AF661189

# *The Complete Book of Yoga*

*KARMA YOGA | BHAKTI YOGA |*
*RĀJA YOGA | JNĀNA YOGA*

*Swami Vivekananda*
Institute of Thought & Philosophy

GRAPEVINE INDIA

Published by

**GRAPEVINE INDIA PUBLISHERS PVT LTD**

www.grapevineindia.com
Delhi | Mumbai
email: grapevineindiapublishers@gmail.com

Ordering Information:
Quantity sales: Special discounts are available on quantity purchases by corporations, associations, and others.
For details, reach out to the publisher.

First published by Grapevine India 2024
Copyright © Grapevine 2024
All rights reserved

The mission of the Institute of Thought and Philosophy is to preserve and propagate the teachings of Swami Vivekananda. This great Indian spiritual leader is known for introducing the West to Hinduism. Drawing from his vast literary legacy, we provide valuable insights and practical guidance for modern living.

Have any query or feedback? Please reach out to us at ITPPress123@gmail.com

# Bhakti

## Definition of Bhakti

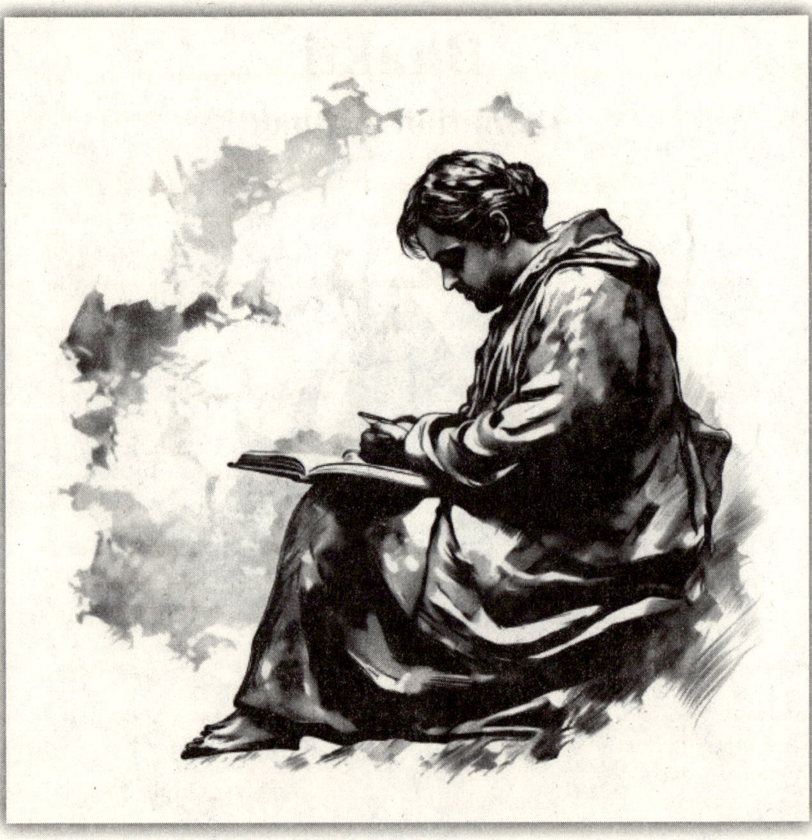

# PRAYER

स तन्मयो ह्यमृत ईशसंस्थो ज्ञः सर्वगो भुवनस्यास्य गोप्ता ।
य ईशोऽस्य जगतो नित्यमेव नान्यो हेतुर्विद्यत ईशनाम ॥
यो ब्रह्माणं विदधाति पूर्वं यो वै वेदांश्च प्रहिणोति तस्मै ।
तं ह देवं आत्मबुद्धिप्रकाशं मुमुक्षुर्वै शरणमहं प्रपद्ये ॥

"He is the Soul of the Universe; He is Immortal; His is the Rulership; He is the All-knowing, the All-pervading, the Protector of the Universe, the Eternal Ruler. None else is there efficient to govern the world eternally. He who at the beginning of creation projected Brahmâ (i.e. the universal consciousness), and who delivered the Vedas unto him — seeking liberation I go for refuge unto that effulgent One, whose light turns the understanding towards the Âtman."

Shvetâshvatara-Upanishad, VI. 17-18.

# DEFINITION OF BHAKTI

Bhakti-Yoga is a real, genuine search after the Lord, a search beginning, continuing, and ending in love. One single moment of the madness of extreme love to God brings us eternal freedom.

"Bhakti", says Nârada in his explanation of the Bhakti-aphorisms, "is intense love to God"; "When a man gets it, he loves all, hates none; he becomes satisfied for ever".

"This love cannot be reduced to any earthly benefit", because so long as worldly desires last, that kind of love does not come; "Bhakti is greater than karma, greater than Yoga, because these are intended for an object in view, while Bhakti is its own fruition, its own means and its own end."

Bhakti has been the one constant theme of our sages. Apart from the special writers on Bhakti, such as Shândilya or Narada, the great commentators on the Vyâsa-Sutras , evidently advocates of knowledge (Jnâna), have also something very suggestive to say about love. Even when the commentator is anxious to explain many, if not all, of the texts so as to make them import a sort of dry knowledge, the Sutras , in the chapter on worship especially, do not lend themselves to be easily manipulated in that fashion.

There is not really so much difference between knowledge (Jnana) and love (Bhakti) as people sometimes imagine. We shall see, as we go on, that in the end they converge and meet at the same point. So also is it with Râja-Yoga, which when pursued as a means to attain liberation, and not (as unfortunately it frequently becomes in the hands of charlatans and mystery-mongers) as an instrument to hoodwink the unwary, leads us also to the same goal.

The one great advantage of Bhakti is that it is the easiest and the most natural way to reach the great divine end in view; its great disadvantage is that in its lower forms it oftentimes degenerates into hideous fanaticism. The fanatical crew in Hinduism, or Mohammedanism, or Christianity, have always been almost exclusively recruited from these worshippers on the lower planes of Bhakti.

That singleness of attachment (Nishthâ) to a loved object, without which no genuine love can grow, is very often also the cause of the denunciation of everything else. All the weak and undeveloped minds in every religion or country have only one way of loving their own ideal, i.e. by hating every other ideal.

Herein is the explanation of why the same man who is so lovingly attached to his own ideal of God, so devoted to his own ideal of religion, becomes a howling fanatic as soon as he sees or hears anything of any other ideal. This kind of love is somewhat like the canine instinct of guarding the master's property from intrusion; only, the instinct of the dog is better than the reason of man, for the dog never mistakes its master for an enemy in whatever dress he may come before it.

Again, the fanatic loses all power of judgment. Personal considerations are in his case of such absorbing interest that to him it is no question at all what a man says — whether it is right or wrong; but the one thing he is always particularly careful to know is who says it. The same man who is kind, good, honest, and loving to people of his own opinion, will not hesitate to do the vilest deeds when they are directed against persons beyond the pale of his own religious brotherhood.

But this danger exists only in that stage of Bhakti which is called thepreparatory (Gauni). When Bhakti has become ripe and has passed into that form which is called the supreme (Parâ), no more is there any fear of these hideous manifestations of fanaticism; that soul which is overpowered by this higher form of Bhakti is too near the God of Love to become an instrument for the diffusion of hatred.

It is not given to all of us to be harmonious in the building up of our characters in this life: yet we know that that character is of the noblest type in which all these three — knowledge and love and Yoga — are harmoniously fused. Three things are necessary for a bird to fly — the two wings and the tail as a rudder for steering. Jnana (Knowledge) is the one wing, Bhakti (Love) is the other, and Yoga is the tail that keeps up the balance.

For those who cannot pursue all these three forms of worship together in harmony and take up, therefore, Bhakti alone as their way, it is necessary always to remember that forms and ceremonials, though absolutely necessary for the progressive soul, have no other value than taking us on to that state in which we feel the most intense love to God.

There is a little difference in opinion between the teachers of knowledge and those of love, though both admit the power of Bhakti. The Jnanis hold Bhakti to be an instrument of liberation, the Bhaktas look upon it both as the instrument and the thing to be attained.

To my mind this is a distinction without much difference. In fact, Bhakti, when used as an instrument, really means a lower form of worship, and the higher form becomes inseparable from the lower form of realisation at a later stage. Each seems to lay a great stress upon his own peculiar method of worship, forgetting that with perfect love true knowledge is bound to come even unsought, and that from perfect knowledge true love is inseparable.

Bearing this in mind let us try to understand what the great Vedantic commentators have to say on the subject. In explaining the Sutra Âvrittirasakridupadeshât (Meditation is necessary, that having been often enjoined.), Bhagavân Shankara says, "Thus people say, 'He is devoted to the king, he is devoted to the Guru'; they say this of him who follows his Guru, and does so, having that following as the one end in view.

Similarly they say, 'The loving wife meditates on her loving husband'; here also a kind of eager and continuous remembrance is meant." This is devotion according to Shankara.

So says Bhagavân Râmânuja in his commentary on the Sutra Athâto Brahma-jijnâsâ:

"Meditation again is a constant remembrance (of the thing meditated upon) flowing like an unbroken stream of oil poured out from one vessel to another. When this kind of remembering has been attained (in relation to God) all bondages break.

"Thus it is spoken of in the scriptures regarding constant remembering as a means to liberation. This remembering again is of the same form as seeing, because it is of the same meaning as in the passage, 'When He who is far and near is seen, the bonds of the heart are broken, all doubts vanish, and all effects of work disappear' He who is near can be seen, but he who is far can only be remembered. Nevertheless the scripture says that he have to see Him who is near as well as Him who, is far, thereby indicating to us that the above kind of remembering is as good as seeing.

"This remembrance when exalted assumes the same form as seeing. Worship is constant remembering as may be seen from the essential texts of scriptures. Knowing, which is the same as repeated worship, has been described as constant remembering.

Thus the memory, which has attained to the height of what is as good as direct perception, is spoken of in the Shruti as a means of liberation.

"This Atman is not to be reached through various sciences, nor by intellect, nor by much study of the Vedas. Whomsoever this Atman desires, by him is the Atman attained, unto him this Atman discovers Himself.

"Here, after saying that mere hearing, thinking and meditating are not the means of attaining this Atman, it is said, 'Whom this Atman desires, by him the Atman is attained.'

"The extremely beloved is desired; by whomsoever this Atman is extremely beloved, he becomes the most beloved of the Atman. So that this beloved may attain the Atman, the Lord Himself helps.

"For it has been said by the Lord: 'Those who are constantly attached to Me and worship Me with love — I give that direction to their will by which they come to Me.'

"Therefore it is said that, to whomsoever this remembering, which is of the same form as direct perception, is very dear, because it is dear to the Object of such memory perception, he is desired by the Supreme Atman, by him the Supreme Atman is attained. This constant remembrance is denoted by the word Bhakti."

In commenting on the Sutra of Patanjali, Ishvara pranidhânâdvâ, i.e. "Or by the worship of the Supreme Lord" — Bhoja says, "Pranidhâna is that sort of Bhakti in which, without seeking results, such as sense-enjoyments etc., all works are dedicated to that Teacher of teachers."

Bhagavan Vyâsa also, when commenting on the same, defines Pranidhana as "the form of Bhakti by which the mercy of the Supreme Lord comes to the Yogi, and blesses him by granting him his desires".

According to Shândilya, "Bhakti is intense love to God." The best definition is, however, that given by the king of Bhaktas, Prahlâda:

या प्रीतिरविवेकानां विषयेष्वनपायिनी ।
त्वामनुस्मरतः सा मे हृदयान्मासर्पतु ॥

"That deathless love which the ignorant have for the fleeting objects of the senses — as I keep meditating on Thee — may not that love slip away from my heart!"

Love ! For whom? For the Supreme Lord Ishvara. Love for any other being, however great cannot be Bhakti; for, as Ramanuja says in his Shri Bhâshya , quoting an ancient Âchârya, i.e. a great teacher:

आब्रह्मस्तम्बपर्यन्ताः जगदन्तर्व्यवस्थिताः ।
प्राणिनः कर्मजनितसंसारवशवर्तिनः ॥
यतस्ततो न ते ध्याने ध्यानिनामुपकारकाः ।
अविद्यान्तर्गतास्सर्वे ते हि संसारगोचराः ॥

"From Brahmâ to a clump of grass, all things that live in the world are slaves of birth and death caused by Karma; therefore they cannot be helpful as objects of meditation, because they are all in ignorance and subject to change."

In commenting on the word Anurakti used by Shandilya, the commentator Svapneshvara says that it means Anu, after, and Rakti, attachment; i.e. the attachment which comes after the knowledge of the nature and glory of God; else a blind attachment to any one, e.g. to wife or children, would be Bhakti. We plainly see, therefore, that Bhakti is a series or succession of mental efforts at religious realisation beginning with ordinary worship and ending in a supreme intensity of love for Ishvara.

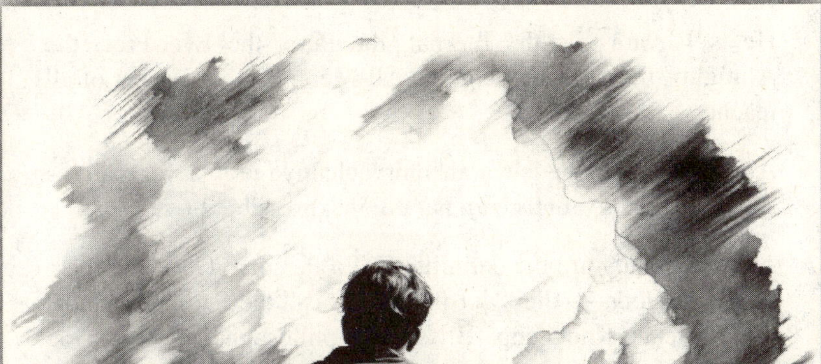

# The Philosophy of Ishvara

Who is Ishvara?

Janmâdyasya yatah — "From whom is the birth, continuation, and dissolution of the universe."

He is Ishvara — "the Eternal, the Pure, the Ever-Free, the Almighty, the All-Knowing, the All-Merciful, the Teacher of all teachers"

And above all, Sa Ishvarah anirvachaniya-premasvarupah — "He the Lord is, of His own nature, inexpressible Love."

These certainly are the definitions of a Personal God. Are there then two Gods — the "Not this, not this," the Sat-chit-ânanda, the Existence-Knowledge-Bliss of the philosopher, and this God of Love of the Bhakta?

No, it is the same Sat-chit-ananda who is also the God of Love, the impersonal and personal in one. It has always to be understood that the Personal God worshipped by the Bhakta is not separate or different from the Brahman. All is Brahman, the One without a second; only the Brahman, as unity or absolute, is too much of an abstraction to be loved and worshipped; so the Bhakta chooses the relative aspect of Brahman, that is, Ishvara, the Supreme Ruler.

To use a simile: Brahman is as the clay or substance out of which an infinite variety of articles are fashioned. As clay, they are all one; but form or manifestation differentiates them. Before every one of them was made, they all existed potentially in the clay, and, of course, they are identical substantially; but when formed, and so long as the form remains, they are separate and different; the clay-mouse can never become a clay-elephant, because, as manifestations, form alone makes them what they are, though as unformed clay they are all one.

Ishvara is the highest manifestation of the Absolute Reality, or in other words, the highest possible reading of the Absolute by the human mind. Creation is eternal, and so also is Ishvara.

In the fourth Pâda of the fourth chapter of his Sutras , after stating the almost infinite power and knowledge which will come to the liberated soul after the attainment of Moksha, Vyâsa makes the remark, in an aphorism, that none, however, will get the power of creating, ruling, and dissolving the universe, because that belongs to God alone.

In explaining the Sutra it is easy for the dualistic commentators to show how it is ever impossible for a subordinate soul, Jiva, to have the infinite power and total independence of God. The thorough dualistic commentator Madhvâchârya deals with this passage in his usual summary method by quoting a verse from the Varâha Purâna.

In explaining this aphorism the commentator Râmânuja says,

"This doubt being raised, whether among the powers of the liberated souls is included that unique power of the Supreme One, that is, of creation etc. of the universe and even the Lordship of all, or whether, without that, the glory of the liberated consists only in the direct perception of the Supreme One, we get as an argument the following: It is reasonable that the liberated get the Lordship of the universe, because the scriptures say, 'He attains to extreme sameness with the Supreme One and all his desires are realised.' Now extreme sameness and realisation of all desires cannot be attained without the unique power of the Supreme Lord, namely, that of governing the universe.

"Therefore, to attain the realisation of all desires and the extreme sameness with the Supreme, we must all admit that the liberated get the power of ruling the whole universe. To this we reply, that the liberated get all the powers except that of ruling the universe. Ruling the universe is guiding the form and the life and the desires of all the sentient and the non-sentient beings. The liberated ones from whom all that veils His true nature has been removed, only enjoy the unobstructed perception of the Brahman, but do not possess the power of ruling the universe.

"This is proved from the scriptural text, "From whom all these things are born, by which all that are born live, unto whom they, departing, return — ask about it. That is Brahman.' If this quality of ruling the universe be a quality common even to the liberated then this text would not apply as a definition of Brahman defining Him through His rulership of the universe. The uncommon attributes alone define a thing; therefore in texts like — 'My beloved boy, alone, in the beginning there existed the One without a second. That saw and felt, "I will give birth to the many." That projected heat.' — 'Brahman indeed alone existed in the beginning. That One evolved. That projected a blessed form, the Kshatra. All these gods are Kshatras: Varuna, Soma, Rudra, Parjanya, Yama, Mrityu, Ishâna.' — 'Atman indeed existed alone in the beginning; nothing else vibrated; He thought of projecting the world; He projected the world after.' — 'Alone Nârâyana existed; neither Brahmâ, nor Ishana, nor the Dyâvâ-Prithivi, nor the stars, nor water, nor fire, nor Soma, nor the sun. He did not take pleasure alone. He after His meditation had one daughter, the ten organs, etc.' — and in others as, 'Who living in the earth is separate from the earth, who living in the Atman, etc.' — the Shrutis speak of the Supreme One as the subject of the work of ruling the universe. . . . Nor in these descriptions of the ruling of the universe is there any position for the liberated soul, by which such a soul may have the ruling of the universe ascribed to it."

In explaining the next Sutra, Ramanuja says, "If you say it is not so, because there are direct texts in the Vedas in evidence to the contrary, these texts refer to the glory of the liberated in the spheres of the subordinate deities." This also is an easy solution of the difficulty. Although the system of Ramanuja admits the unity of the total, within that totality of existence there are, according to him, eternal differences. Therefore, for all practical purposes, this system also being dualistic, it was easy for Ramanuja to keep the distinction between the personal soul and the Personal God very clear.

We shall now try to understand what the great representative of the Advaita School has to say on the point. We shall see how the Advaita system maintains all the hopes and aspirations of the dualist intact, and at the same time propounds its own solution of the problem in consonance with the high destiny of divine humanity.

Those who aspire to retain their individual mind even after liberation and to remain distinct will have ample opportunity of realising their aspirations and enjoying the blessing of the qualified Brahman. These are they who have been spoken of in the Bhâgavata Purâna thus: "O king, such are the, glorious qualities of the Lord that the sages whose only pleasure is in the Self, and from whom all fetters have fallen off, even they love the Omnipresent with the love that is for love's sake."

These are they who are spoken of by the Sânkhyas as getting merged in nature in this cycle, so that, after attaining perfection, they may come out in the next as lords of world-systems. But none of these ever becomes equal to God (Ishvara).

Those who attain to that state where there is neither creation, nor created, nor creator, where there is neither knower, nor knowable, nor knowledge, where there is neither I, nor thou, nor he, where there is neither subject, nor object, nor relation, "there, who is seen by whom?" — such persons have gone beyond everything to "where words cannot go nor mind", gone to that which the Shrutis declare as "Not this, not this". But for those who cannot, or will not reach this state, there will inevitably remain the triune vision of the one undifferentiated Brahman as nature, soul, and the interpenetrating sustainer of both — Ishvara.

So, when Prahlâda forgot himself, he found neither the universe nor its cause; all was to him one Infinite, undifferentiated by name and form; but as soon as he remembered that he was Prahlada, there was the universe before him and with it the Lord of the universe — "the Repository of an infinite number of blessed qualities".

So it was with the blessed Gopis. So long as they had lost sense of their own personal identity and individuality, they were all

Krishnas, and when they began again to think of Him as the One to be worshipped, then they were Gopis again, and immediately

तासामाविरभूच्छौरिः स्मयमानमुखाम्बुजः ।
पीताम्बरधरः स्रग्वी साक्षान्मन्मथमन्मथः ॥

"Unto them appeared Krishna with a smile on His lotus face, clad in yellow robes and having garlands on, the embodied conqueror (in beauty) of the god of love."

Now to go back to our Acharya Shankara: "Those", he says, "who by worshipping the qualified Brahman attain conjunction with the Supreme Ruler, preserving their own mind — is their glory limited or unlimited? This doubt arising, we get as an argument: Their glory should be unlimited because of the scriptural texts, 'They attain their own kingdom', 'To him all the gods offer worship', 'Their desires are fulfilled in all the worlds'. As an answer to this, Vyasa writes, 'Without the power of ruling the universe.' Barring the power of creation etc. of the universe, the other powers such as Animâ etc. are acquired by the liberated. As to ruling the universe, that belongs to the eternally perfect Ishvara. Why? Because He is the subject of all the scriptural texts as regards creation etc., and the liberated souls are not mentioned therein in any connection whatsoever. The Supreme Lord indeed is alone engaged in ruling the universe. The texts as to creation etc. all point to Him. Besides, there is given the adjective 'ever-perfect'. Also the scriptures say that the powers Anima etc. of the others are from the search after and the worship of God. Therefore they have no place in the ruling of the universe. Again, on account of their possessing their own minds, it is possible that their wills may differ, and that, whilst one desires creation, another may desire destruction. The only way of avoiding this conflict is to make all wills subordinate to some one will. Therefore the conclusion is that the wills of the liberated are dependent on the will of the Supreme Ruler."

Bhakti, then, can be directed towards Brahman, only in His personal aspect. — "The way is more difficult for those whose mind is attached to the Absolute!" Bhakti has to float on smoothly with the current of our nature. True it is that we cannot have; any idea of the Brahman which is not anthropomorphic, but is it not equally true of everything we know? The greatest psychologist the world has ever known, Bhagavan Kapila, demonstrated ages ago that human consciousness is one of the elements in the make-up of all the objects of our perception and conception, internal as well as external. Beginning with our bodies and going up to Ishvara, we may see that every object of our perception is this consciousness plus something else, whatever that may be; and this unavoidable mixture is what we ordinarily think of as reality. Indeed it is, and ever will be, all of the reality that is possible for the human mind to know. Therefore to say that Ishvara is unreal, because He is anthropomorphic, is sheer nonsense. It sounds very much like the occidentals squabble on idealism and realism, which fearful-looking quarrel has for its foundation a mere play on the word "real". The idea of Ishvara covers all the ground ever denoted and connoted by the word real, and Ishvara is as real as anything else in the universe; and after all, the word real means nothing more than what has now been pointed out. Such is our philosophical conception of Ishvara.

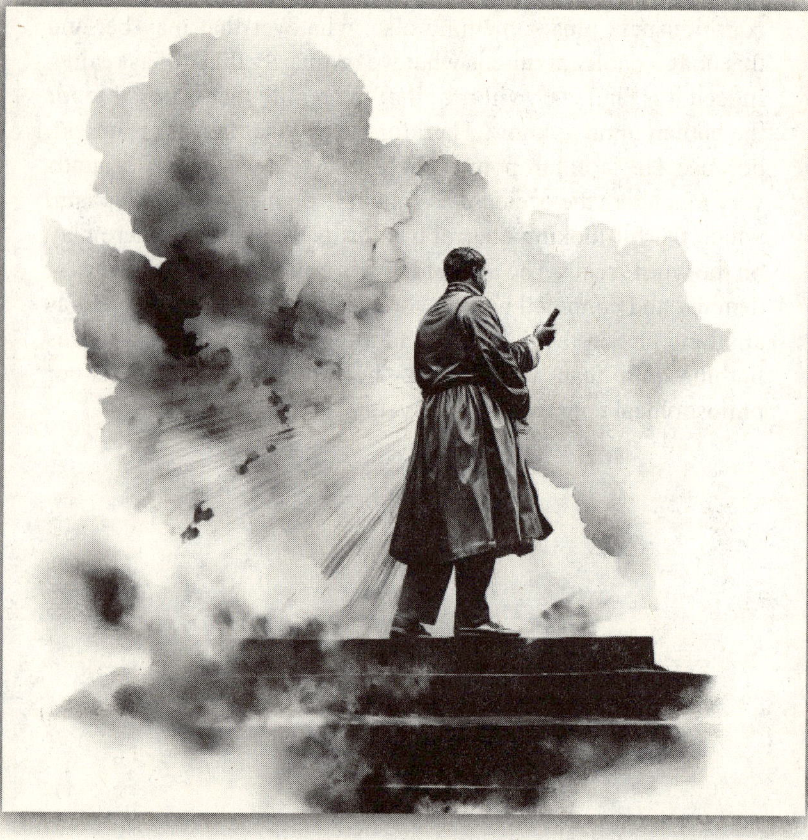

# Spiritual Realisation, The Aim of Bhakti-Yoga

To the Bhakta these dry details are necessary only to strengthen his will; beyond that they are of no use to him. For he is treading on a path which is fitted very soon to lead him beyond the hazy and turbulent regions of reason, to lead him to the realm of realisation.

He, soon, through the mercy of the Lord, reaches a plane where pedantic and powerless reason is left far behind, and the mere intellectual groping through the dark gives place to the daylight of direct perception. He no more reasons and believes, he almost perceives. He no more argues, he senses.

And is not this seeing God, and feeling God, and enjoying God higher than everything else? Nay, Bhaktas have not been wanting who have maintained that it is higher than even Moksha — liberation. And is it not also the highest utility?

There are people — and a good many of them too — in the world who are convinced that only that is of use and utility which brings to man creature-comforts. Even religion, God, eternity, soul, none of these is of any use to them, as they do not bring them money or physical comfort. To such, all those things which do not go to gratify the senses and appease the appetites are of no utility.

In every mind, utility, however, is conditioned by its own peculiar wants. To men, therefore, who never rise higher than eating, drinking, begetting progeny, and dying, the only gain is in sense enjoyments; and they must wait and go through many more births and reincarnations to learn to feel even the faintest necessity for anything higher.

But those to whom the eternal interests of the soul are of much higher value than the fleeting interests of this mundane life, to whom the gratification of the senses is but like the thoughtless play of the baby, to them God and the love of God form the highest and the only utility of human existence. Thank God there are some such still living in this world of too much worldliness.

Bhakti-Yoga, as we have said, is divided into the Gauni or the preparatory, and the Parâ or the supreme forms. We shall find, as we go on, how in the preparatory stage we unavoidably stand in need of many concrete helps to enable us to get on; and indeed the mythological and symbological parts of all religions are natural growths which early environ the aspiring soul and help it Godward.

It is also a significant fact that spiritual giants have been produced only in those systems of religion where there is an exuberant growth of rich mythology and ritualism. The dry fanatical forms of religion which attempt to eradicate all that is poetical, all that is beautiful and sublime, all that gives a firm grasp to the infant mind tottering in its Godward way — the forms which attempt to break down the very ridge-poles of the spiritual roof, and in their ignorant and superstitious conceptions of truth try to drive away all that is life-giving, all that furnishes the formative material to the spiritual plant growing in the human soul — such forms of religion too soon find that all that is left to them is but an empty shell, a contentless frame of words and sophistry with perhaps a little flavour of a kind of social scavengering or the so-called spirit of reform.

The vast mass of those whose religion is like this, are conscious or unconscious materialists — the end and aim of their lives here and hereafter being enjoyment, which indeed is to them the alpha and the omega of human life, and which is their Ishtâpurta. Work like street-cleaning and scavengering, intended for the material comfort of man is, according to them, the be-all and end-all of human existence; and the sooner the followers of this curious mixture of ignorance and fanaticism come out in their true colours and join, as they well deserve to do, the ranks of atheists and materialists, the better will it be for the world.

One ounce of the practice of righteousness and of spiritual Self-realisation outweighs tons and tons of frothy talk and nonsensical sentiments. Show us one, but one gigantic spiritual genius growing out of all this dry dust of ignorance and fanaticism; and if you cannot, close your mouths, open the windows of your hearts to the clear light of truth, and sit like children at the feet of those who know what they are talking about — the sages of India. Let us then listen attentively to what they say.

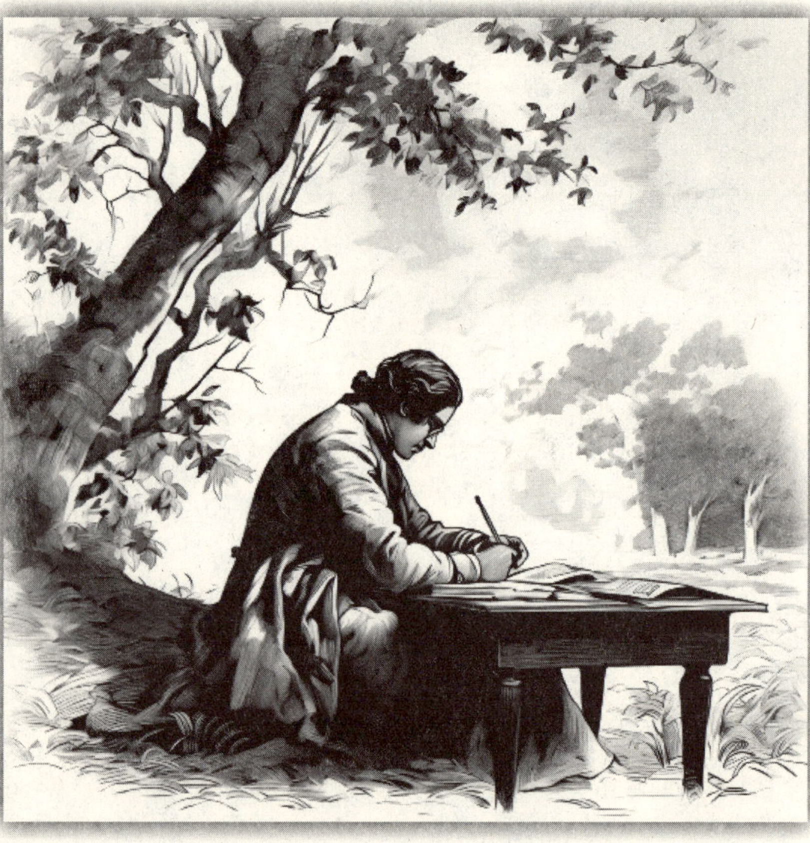

# The Method and The Means

In regard to the method and the means of Bhakti-Yoga we read in the commentary of Bhagavan Ramanuja on the Vedanta-Sutras: "The attaining of That comes through discrimination, controlling the passions, practice, sacrificial work, purity, strength, and suppression of excessive joy."

Viveka or discrimination is, according to Ramanuja, discriminating, among other things, the pure food from the impure. According to him, food becomes impure from three causes: (1) by the nature of the food itself, as in the case of garlic etc.; (2) owing to its coming from wicked and accursed persons; and (3) from physical impurities, such as dirt, or hair, etc.

The Shrutis say, When the food is pure, the Sattva element gets purified, and the memory becomes unwavering", and Ramanuja quotes this from the Chhândogya Upanishad.

The question of food has always been one of the most vital with the Bhaktas. Apart from the extravagance into which some of the Bhakti sects have run, there is a great truth underlying this question of food.

We must remember that, according to the Sankhya philosophy, the Sattva, Rajas, and Tamas, which in the state of homogeneous equilibrium form the Prakriti, and in the heterogeneous disturbed condition form the universe — are both the substance and the quality of Prakriti. As such they are the materials out of which every human form has been manufactured, and the predominance of the Sattva material is what is absolutely necessary for spiritual development.

The materials which we receive through our food into our body-structure go a great way to determine our mental constitution; therefore the food we eat has to be particularly taken care of. However, in this matter, as in others, the fanaticism into which the disciples invariably fall is not to be laid at the door of the masters.

And this discrimination of food is, after all, of secondary importance. The very same passage quoted above is explained by Shankara in his Bhâshya on the Upanishads in a different way by giving an entirely different meaning to the word Âhâra, translated generally as food.

According to him, “That which is gathered in is Ahara. The knowledge of the sensations, such as sound etc., is gathered in for the enjoyment of the enjoyer (self); the purification of the knowledge which gathers in the perception of the senses is the purifying of the food (Ahara). The word ‘purification-of-food’ means the acquiring of the knowledge of sensations untouched by the defects of attachment, aversion, and delusion; such is the meaning. Therefore such knowledge or Ahara being purified, the Sattva material of the possessor it — the internal organ — will become purified, and the Sattva being purified, an unbroken memory of the Infinite One, who has been known in His real nature from scriptures, will result.”

These two explanations are apparently conflicting, yet both are true and necessary. The manipulating and controlling of what may be called the finer body, viz the mood, are no doubt higher functions than the controlling of the grosser body of flesh. But the control of the grosser is absolutely necessary to enable one to arrive at the control of the finer.

The beginner, therefore, must pay particular attention to all such dietetic rules as have come down from the line of his accredited teachers; but the extravagant, meaningless fanaticism, which has driven religion entirely to the kitchen, as may be noticed in the case of many of our sects, without any hope of the noble truth of that religion ever coming out to the sunlight of spirituality, is a peculiar sort of pure and simple materialism.

It is neither Jnâna, nor Bhakti, nor Karma; it is a special kind of lunacy, and those who pin their souls to it are more likely to go to lunatic asylums than to Brahmaloka. So it stands to reason that discrimination in the choice of food is necessary for the attainment of this higher state of mental composition which cannot be easily obtained otherwise.

Controlling the passions is the next thing to be attended to. To restrain the Indriyas (organs) from going towards the objects of the senses, to control them and bring them under the guidance of the will, is the very central virtue in religious culture.

Then comes the practice of self-restraint and self-denial. All the immense possibilities of divine realisation in the soul cannot get actualised without struggle and without such practice on the part of the aspiring devotee. "The mind must always think of the Lord."

It is very hard at first to compel the mind to think of the Lord always, but with every new effort the power to do so grows stronger in us. "By practice, O son of Kunti, and by non-attachment is it attained", says Shri Krishna in the Gita.

And then as to sacrificial work, it is understood that the five great sacrificed (To gods, sages, manes, guests, and all creatures.) (Panchamahâyajna) have to be performed as usual.

Purity is absolutely the basic work, the bed-rock upon which the whole Bhakti-building rests. Cleansing the external body and discriminating the food are both easy, but without internal cleanliness and purity, these external observances are of no value whatsoever.

In the list of qualities conducive to purity, as given by Ramanuja, there are enumerated, Satya, truthfulness; Ârjava, sincerity; Dayâ, doing good to others without any gain to one's self; Ahimsâ, not injuring others by thought, word, or deed; Anabhidhyâ, not coveting others' goods, not thinking vain thoughts, and not brooding over injuries received from another.

In this list, the one idea that deserves special notice is Ahimsa, non-injury to others. This duty of non-injury is, so to speak, obligatory on us in relation to all beings. As with some, it does not simply mean the non-injuring of human beings and mercilessness towards the lower animals; nor, as with some others, does it mean the protecting of cats and dogs and feeding of ants with sugar — with liberty to injure brother-man in every horrible way! It is remarkable that almost every good idea in this world can be carried to a disgusting extreme.

A good practice carried to an extreme and worked in accordance with the letter of the law becomes a positive evil. The stinking monks of certain religious sects, who do not bathe lest the vermin on their bodies should be killed, never think of the discomfort and disease they bring to their fellow human beings. They do not, however, belong to the religion of the Vedas!

The test of Ahimsa is absence of jealousy. Any man may do a good deed or make a good gift on the spur of the moment or under the pressure of some superstition or priestcraft; but the real lover of mankind is he who is jealous of none. The so-called great men of the world may all be seen to become jealous of each other for a small name, for a little fame, and for a few bits of gold. So long as this jealousy exists in a heart, it is far away from the perfection of Ahimsa.

The cow does not eat meat, nor does the sheep. Are they great Yogis, great non-injurers (Ahimsakas)? Any fool may abstain from eating this or that; surely that gives him no more distinction than to herbivorous animals.

The man who will mercilessly cheat widows and orphans and do the vilest deeds for money is worse than any brute even if he lives entirely on grass. The man whose heart never cherishes even the thought of injury to any one, who rejoices at the prosperity of even his greatest enemy, that man is the Bhakta, he is the Yogi, he is the Guru of all, even though he lives every day of his life on the flesh of swine.

Therefore we must always remember that external practices have value only as helps to develop internal purity. It is better to have internal purity alone when minute attention to external observances is not practicable. But woe unto the man and woe unto the nation that forgets the real, internal, spiritual essentials of religion and mechanically clutches with death-like grasp at all external forms and never lets them go. The forms have value only so far as they are expressions of the life within. If they have ceased to express life, crush them out without mercy.

The next means to the attainment of Bhakti-Yoga is strength (Anavasâda). "This Atman is not to be attained by the weak", says the Shruti. Both physical weakness and mental weakness are meant here. "The strong, the hardy" are the only fit students.

What can puny, little, decrepit things do? They will break to pieces whenever the mysterious forces of the body and mind are even slightly awakened by the practice of any of the Yogas. It is "the young, the healthy, the strong" that can score success.

Physical strength, therefore, is absolutely necessary. It is the strong body alone that can bear the shock of reaction resulting from the attempt to control the organs. He who wants to become a Bhakta must be strong, must be healthy. When the miserably weak attempt any of the Yogas, they are likely to get some incurable malady, or they weaken their minds. Voluntarily weakening the body is really no prescription for spiritual enlightenment.

The mentally weak also cannot succeed in attaining the Atman. The person who aspires to be a Bhakta must be cheerful. In the Western world the idea of a religious man is that he never smiles, that a dark cloud must always hang over his face, which, again, must be long drawn with the jaws almost collapsed. People with emaciated bodies and long faces are fit subjects for the physician, they are not Yogis. It is the cheerful mind that is persevering. It is the strong mind that hews its way through a thousand difficulties. And this, the hardest task of all, the cutting of our way out of the net of Maya, is the work reserved only for giant wills.

Yet at the same time excessive mirth should be avoided (Anuddharsha). Excessive mirth makes us unfit for serious thought. It also fritters away the energies of the mind in vain. The stronger the will, the less the yielding to the sway of the emotions. Excessive hilarity is quite as objectionable as too much of sad seriousness, and all religious realisation is possible only when the mind is in a steady, peaceful condition of harmonious equilibrium.

It is thus that one may begin to learn how to love the Lord.

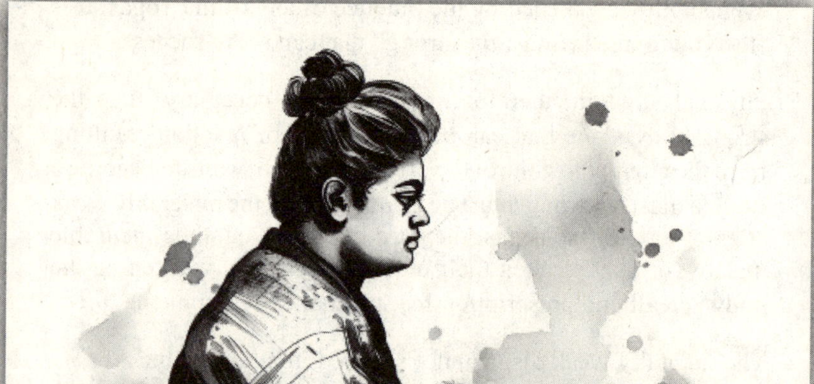

# The Preparation

The best definition given of Bhakti-Yoga is perhaps embodied in the verse: "May that love undying which the non-discriminating have for the fleeting objects of the senses never leave this heart of mine — of me who seek after Thee!"

We see what a strong love men, who do not know any better, have for sense-objects, for money, dress, their wives, children, friends, and possessions. What a tremendous clinging they have to all these things! So in the above prayer the sage says, "I will have that attachment, that tremendous clinging, only to Thee."

This love, when given to God, is called Bhakti. Bhakti is not destructive; it teaches us that no one of the faculties we have has been given in vain, that through them is the natural way to come to liberation. Bhakti does not kill out our tendencies, it does not go against nature, but only gives it a higher and more powerful direction.

How naturally we love objects of the senses! We cannot but do so, because they are so real to us. We do not ordinarily see anything real about higher things, but when a man has seen something real beyond the senses, beyond the universe of senses, the idea is that he can have a strong attachment, only it should be transferred to the object beyond the senses, which is God. And when the same kind of love that has before been given to sense-objects is given to God, it is called Bhakti. According to the sage Râmânuja, the following are the preparations for getting that intense love.

The first is Viveka. It is a very curious thing, especially to people of the West. It means, according to Ramanuja, "discrimination of food". Food contains all the energies that go to make up the forces of our body and mind; it has been transferred, and conserved, and given new directions in my body, but my body and mind have nothing essentially different from the food that I ate.

Just as the force and matter we find in the material world become body and mind in us, so, essentially, the difference between body and mind and the food we eat is only in manifestation. It being so, that out of the material particles of our food we construct the instrument of thought, and that from the finer forces lodged in these particles we manufacture thought itself, it naturally follows, that both this thought and the instrument will be modified by the food we take.

There are certain kinds of food that produce a certain change in the mind; we see it every day. There are other sorts which produce a change in the body, and in the long run have a tremendous effect on the mind. It is a great thing to learn; a good deal of the misery we suffer is occasioned by the food we take.

You find that after a heavy and indigestible meal it is very hard to control the mind; it is running, running all the time. There are certain foods which are exciting; if you eat such food, you find that you cannot control the mind. It is obvious that after drinking a large quantity of wine, or other alcoholic beverage, a man finds that his mind would not be controlled; it runs away from his control.

According to Ramanuja, there are three things in food we must avoid. First, there is Jâti, the nature, or species of the food, that must be considered. All exciting food should be avoided, as meat, for instance; this should not be taken because it is by its very nature impure.

We can get it only by taking the life of another. We get pleasure for a moment, and another creature has to give up its life to give us that pleasure. Not only so, but we demoralise other human beings. It would be rather better if every man who eats meat killed the animal himself; but, instead of doing so, society gets a class of persons to do that business for them, for doing which, it hates them.

In England no butcher can serve on a jury, the idea being that he is cruel by nature. Who makes him cruel? Society. If we did not eat beef and mutton, there would be no butchers. Eating meat is only allowable for people who do very hard work, and who are not going to be Bhaktas; but if you are going to be Bhaktas, you should avoid meat. Also, all exciting foods, such as onions, garlic, and all evil-smelling food, as "sauerkraut". Any food that has been standing for days, till its condition is changed, any food whose natural juices have been almost dried ups any food that is malodorous, should be avoided.

The next thing that is to be considered as regards food is still more intricate to Western minds — it is what is called Âshraya, i.e. the person from whom it comes.

This is rather a mysterious theory of the Hindus. The idea is that each man has a certain aura round him, and whatever thing he touches, a part of his character, as it were, his influence, is left on it. It is supposed that a man's character emanates from him, as it were, like a physical force, and whatever he touches is affected by it.

So we must take care who touches our food when it is cooked; a wicked or immoral person must not touch it. One who wants to be a Bhakta must not dine with people whom he knows to be very wicked, because their infection will come through the food.

The other form of purity to be observed is Nimitta, or instruments. Dirt and dust must not be in food. Food should not be brought from the market and placed on the table unwashed. We must be careful also about the saliva and other secretions.

The lips ought never, for instance, to be touched with the fingers. The mucous membrane is the most delicate part of the body, and all tendencies are conveyed very easily by the saliva. Its contact, therefore, is to be regarded as not only offensive, but dangerous. Again, we must not eat food, half of which has been eaten by someone else. When these things are avoided in food, it becomes pure; pure food brings a pure mind, and in a pure mind is a constant memory of God.

Let me tell you the same thing as explained by another commentator, Shankarâchârya, who takes quite another view.

This word for food, in Sanskrit, is derived from the root, meaning to gather. Âhâra means "gathered in".

What is his explanation? He says, the passage that when food is pure the mind will become pure really means that lest we become subject to the senses we should avoid the following: First as to attachment; we must not be extremely attached to anything excepting God. See everything, do everything, but be not attached. As soon as extreme attachment comes, a man loses himself, he is no more master of himself, he is a slave.

If a woman is tremendously attached to a man, she becomes a slave to that man. There is no use in being a slave. There are higher things in this world than becoming a slave to a human being. Love and do good to everybody, but do not become a slave.

In the first place, attachment degenerates us, individually, and in the second place, makes us extremely selfish. Owing to this failing, we want to injure others to do good to those we love. A good many of the wicked deeds done in this world are really done through attachment to certain persons. So all attachment excepting that for good works should be avoided; but love should be given to everybody.

Then as to jealousy. There should be no jealousy in regard to objects of the senses; jealousy is the root of all evil, and a most difficult thing to conquer.

Next, delusion. We always take one thing for another, and act upon that, with the result that we bring misery upon ourselves. We take the bad for the good. Anything that titillates our nerves for a moment we think; as the highest good, and plunge into it immediately, but find, when it is too late, that it has given us a tremendous blow. Every day, we run into this error, and we often continue in it all our lives.

When the senses, without being extremely attached, without jealousy, or without delusion, work in the world, such work or collection of impressions is called pure food, according to

Shankaracharya. When pure food is taken, the mind is able to take in objects and think about them without attachment, jealousy or delusion; then the mind becomes pure, and then there is constant memory of God in that mind.

It is quite natural for one to say that Shankara's meaning is the best, but I wish to add that one should not neglect Ramanuja's interpretation either. It is only when you take care of the real material food that the rest will come. It is very true that mind is the master, but very few of us are not bound by the senses. We are all controlled by matter; and as long as we are so controlled, we must take material aids; and then, when we have become strong, we can eat or drink anything we like.

We have to follow Ramanuja in taking care about food and drink; at the same time we must also take care about our mental food. It is very easy to take care about material food, but mental work must go along with it; then gradually our spiritual self will become stronger and stronger, and the physical self less assertive. Then will food hurt you no more.

The great danger is that every man wants to jump at the highest ideal, but jumping is not the way. That ends only in a fall. We are bound down here, and we have to break our chains slowly. This is called Viveka, discrimination.

The next is called Vimoka, freedom from desires. He who wants to love God must get rid of extreme desires, desire nothing except God. This world is good so far as it helps one to go to the higher world. The objects of the senses are good so far as they help us to attain higher objects.

We always forget that this world is a means to an end, and not an end itself. If this were the end we should be immortal here in our physical body; we should never die. But we see people every moment dying around us, and yet, foolishly, we think we shall never die; and from that conviction we come to think that this life is the goal. That is the case with ninety-nine per cent of us.

This notion should be given up at once. This world is good so far as it is a means to perfect ourselves; and as soon as it has ceased to be so, it is evil. So wife, husband, children, money and learning, are good so long as they help us forward; but as soon as they cease to do that, they are nothing but evil.

If the wife help us to attain God, she is a good wife; so with a husband or a child. If money help a man to do good to others, it is of some value; but if not, it is simply a mass of evil, and the sooner it is got rid of, the better.

The next is Abhyâsa, practice. The mind should always go towards God. No other things have any right to withhold it. It should continuously think of God, though this is a very hard task; yet it can be done by persistent practice.

What we are now is the result of our past practice. Again, practice makes us what we shall be. So practice the other way; one sort of turning round has brought us this way, turn the other way and get out of it as soon as you can.

Thinking of the senses has brought us down here — to cry one moment, to rejoice the next, to be at the mercy of every breeze, slave to everything. This is shameful, and yet we call ourselves spirits. Go the other way, think of God; let the mind not think of any physical or mental enjoyment, but of God alone. When it tries to think of anything else, give it a good blow, so that it may turn round and think of God.

As oil poured from one vessel to another falls in an unbroken line, as chimes coming from a distance fall upon the ear as one continuous sound, so should the mind flow towards God in one continuous stream. We should not only impose this practice on the mind, but the senses too should be employed. Instead of hearing foolish things, we must hear about God; instead of talking foolish words, we must talk of God. Instead of reading foolish books, we must read good ones which tell of God.

The greatest aid to this practice of keeping God in memory is, perhaps, music. The Lord says to Nârada, the great teacher of Bhakti, "I do not live in heaven, nor do I live in the heart of the

Yogi, but where My devotees sing My praise, there am I".

Music has such tremendous power over the human mind; it brings it to concentration in a moment. You will find the dull, ignorant, low, brute-like human beings, who never steady their mind for a moment at other times, when they hear attractive music, immediately become charmed and concentrated. Even the minds of animals, such as dogs, lions, cats, and serpents, become charmed with music.

The next is Kriyâ, work — doing good to others. The memory of God will not come to the selfish man. The more we come out and do good to others, the more our hearts will be purified, and God will be in them. According to our scriptures, there are five sorts of work, called the fivefold sacrifice.

First, study. A man must study every day something holy and good. Second, worship of God, angels, or saints, as it may be. Third, our duty to our forefathers.

Fourth, our duty to human beings. Man has no right to live in a house himself, until he builds for the poor also, or for anybody who needs it. The householder's house should be open to everybody that is poor and suffering; then he is a real householder. If he builds a house only for himself and his wife to enjoy, he will never be a lover of God. No man has the right to cook food only for himself; it is for others, and he should have what remains.

It is a common practice in India that when the season's produce first comes into the market, such as strawberries or mangoes, a man buys some of them and gives to the poor. Then he eats of them; and it is a very good example to follow in this country. This training will make a man unselfish, and at the same time, be an excellent object-lesson to his wife and children.

The Hebrews in olden times used to give the first fruits to God. The first of everything should go to the poor; we have only a right to what remains. The poor are God's representatives; anyone that suffers is His representative. Without giving, he who eats and enjoys eating, enjoys sin.

Fifth, our duty to the lower animals. It is diabolical to say that all animals are created for men to be killed and used in any way man likes. It is the devil's gospel, not God's. Think how diabolical it is to cut them up to see whether a nerve quivers or not, in a certain part of the body.

I am glad that in our country such things are not countenanced by the Hindus, whatever encouragement they may get from the foreign government they are under. One portion of the food cooked in a household belongs to the animals also. They should be given food every day; there ought to be hospitals in every city in this country for poor, lame, or blind horses, cows, dogs, and cats, where they should be fed and taken care of.

Then there is Kalyâna, purity, which comprises the following: Satya, truthfulness. He who is true, unto him the God of truth comes. Thought, word, and deed should be perfectly true.

Next Ârjava, straightforwardness, rectitude. The word means, to be simple, no crookedness in the heart, no double-dealing. Even if it is a little harsh, go straightforward, and not crookedly.

Dayâ, pity, compassion. Ahimsâ, not injuring any being by thought, word, or deed.

Dâna, charity. There is no higher virtue than charity. The lowest man is he whose hand draws in, in receiving; and he is the highest man whose hand goes out in giving. The hand was made to give always. Give the last bit of bread you have even if you are starving. You will be free in a moment if you starve yourself to death by giving to another. Immediately you will be perfect, you will become God.

People who have children are bound already. They cannot give away. They want to enjoy their children, and they must pay for it. Are there not enough children in the world? It is only selfishness which says, "I'll have a child for myself".

The next is Anavasâda — not desponding, cheerfulness. Despondency is not religion, whatever else it may be. By being pleasant always and smiling, it takes you nearer to God, nearer than any prayer. How can those minds that are gloomy and dull love? If they talk of love, it is false; they want to hurt others.

Think of the fanatics; they make the longest faces, and all their religion is to fight against others in word and act. Think of what they have done in the past, and of what they would do now if they were given a free hand. They would deluge the whole world in blood tomorrow if it would bring them power. By worshipping power and making long faces, they lose every bit of love from their hearts.

So the man who always feels miserable will never come to God. It is not religion, it is diabolism to say, "I am so miserable." Every man has his own burden to bear. If you are miserable, try to be happy, try to conquer it.

God is not to be reached by the weak. Never be weak. You must be strong; you have infinite strength within you. How else will you conquer anything? How else will you come to God?

At the same time you must avoid excessive merriment, Uddharsha, as it is called. A mind in that state never becomes calm; it becomes fickle. Excessive merriment will always be followed by sorrow. Tears and laughter are near kin. People so often run from one extreme to the other. Let the mind be cheerful, but calm. Never let it run into excesses, because every excess will be followed by a reaction.

These, according to Ramanuja, are the preparations for Bhakti.

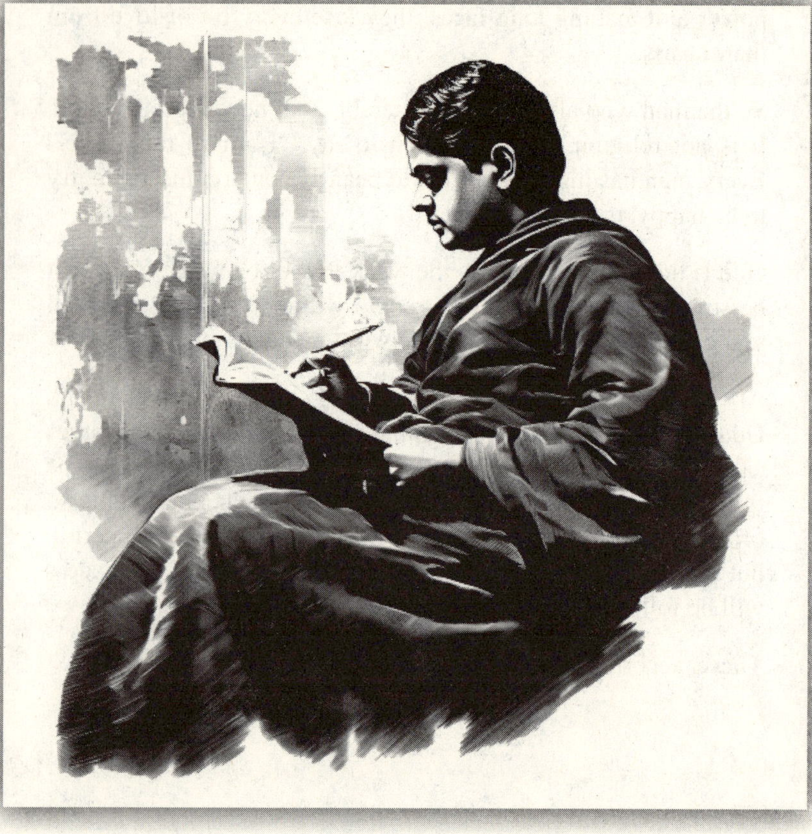

# The Preparatory Renunciation

We have now finished the consideration of what may be called the preparatory Bhakti, and are entering on the study of the Parâ-Bhakti or supreme devotion. We have to speak of a preparation to the practice of this Para-Bhakti. All such preparations are intended only for the purification of the soul.

The repetition of names, the rituals, the forms, and the symbols, all these various things are for the purification of the soul. The greatest purifier among all such things, a purifier without which no one can enter the regions of this higher devotion (Para-Bhakti), is renunciation.

This frightens many; yet, without it, there cannot be any spiritual growth. In all our Yogas this renunciation is necessary. This is the stepping-stone and the real centre and the real heart of all spiritual culture — renunciation. This is religion — renunciation.

When the human soul draws back from the things of the world and tries to go into deeper things; when man, the spirit which has here somehow become concretised and materialised, understands that he is thereby going to be destroyed and to be reduced almost into mere matter, and turns his face away from matter — then begins renunciation, then begins real spiritual growth. The Karma-Yogi's renunciation is in the shape of giving up all the fruits of his action; he is not attached to the results of his labour; he does not care for any reward here or hereafter.

The Râja-Yogi knows that the whole of nature is intended for the soul to acquire experience, and that the result of all the experiences of the soul is for it to become aware of its eternal separateness from nature. The human soul has to understand and realise that it has been spirit, and not matter, through eternity, and that this conjunction of it with matter is and can be only for a time. The Raja-Yogi learns the lesson of renunciation through his own experience of nature.

The Jnâna-Yogi has the harshest of all renunciations to go through, as he has to realise from the very first that the whole of this solid-looking nature is all an illusion. He has to understand that all that is any kind of manifestation of power in nature belongs to the soul, and not to nature. He has to know from the very start that all knowledge and all experience are in the soul and not in nature; so he has at once and by the sheer force of rational conviction to tear himself away from all bondage to nature. He lets nature and all that belongs to her go, he lets them vanish and tries to stand alone!

Of all renunciations, the most natural, so to say, is that of the Bhakti-Yogi. Here there is no violence, nothing to give up, nothing to tear off, as it were, from ourselves, nothing from which we have violently to separate ourselves. The Bhakta's renunciation is easy, smooth flowing, and as natural as the things around us. We see the manifestation of this sort of renunciation, although more or less in the form of caricatures, every day around us.

A man begins to love a woman; after a while he loves another, and the first woman he lets go. She drops out of his mind smoothly, gently, without his feeling the want of her at all. A woman loves a man; she then begins to love another man, and the first one drops off from her mind quite naturally. A man loves his own city, then he begins to love his country, and the intense love for his little city drops off smoothly, naturally.

Again, a man learns to love the whole world; his love for his country, his intense, fanatical patriotism drops off without hurting him, without any manifestation of violence. An uncultured man loves the pleasures of the senses intensely; as he becomes cultured, he begins to love intellectual pleasures, and his sense-enjoyments become less and less.

No man can enjoy a meal with the same gusto or pleasure as a dog or a wolf, but those pleasures which a man gets from intellectual experiences and achievements, the dog can never enjoy. At first, pleasure is in association with the lowest senses; but as soon as an animal reaches a higher plane of existence, the lower kind of pleasures becomes less intense. In human society, the nearer the man is to the animal, the stronger is his pleasure in the senses; and the higher and the more cultured the man is, the greater is his pleasure in intellectual and such other finer pursuits.

So when a man gets even higher than the plane of the intellect, higher than that of mere thought, when he gets to the plane of spirituality and of divine inspiration, he finds there a state of bliss, compared with which all the pleasures of the senses, or even of the intellect, are as nothing. When the moon shines brightly, all the stars become dim; and when the sun shines, the moon herself becomes dim.

The renunciation necessary for the attainment of Bhakti is not obtained by killing anything, but just comes in as naturally as in the presence of an increasingly stronger light, the less intense ones become dimmer and dimmer until they vanish away completely. So this love of the pleasures of the senses and of the intellect is all made dim and thrown aside and cast into the shade by the love of God Himself.

That love of God grows and assumes a form which is called Para-Bhakti or supreme devotion. Forms vanish, rituals fly away, books are superseded; images, temples, churches, religions and sects, countries and nationalities — all these little limitations and bondages fall off by their own nature from him who knows this love of God. Nothing remains to bind him or fetter his freedom. A ship, all of a sudden, comes near a magnetic rock, and its iron bolts and bars are all attracted and drawn out, and the planks get loosened and freely float on the water. Divine grace thus loosens the binding bolts and bars of the soul, and it becomes free.

So in this renunciation auxiliary to devotion, there is no harshness, no dryness no struggle, nor repression nor suppression. The Bhakta has not to suppress any single one of his emotions, he only strives to intensify them and direct them to God.

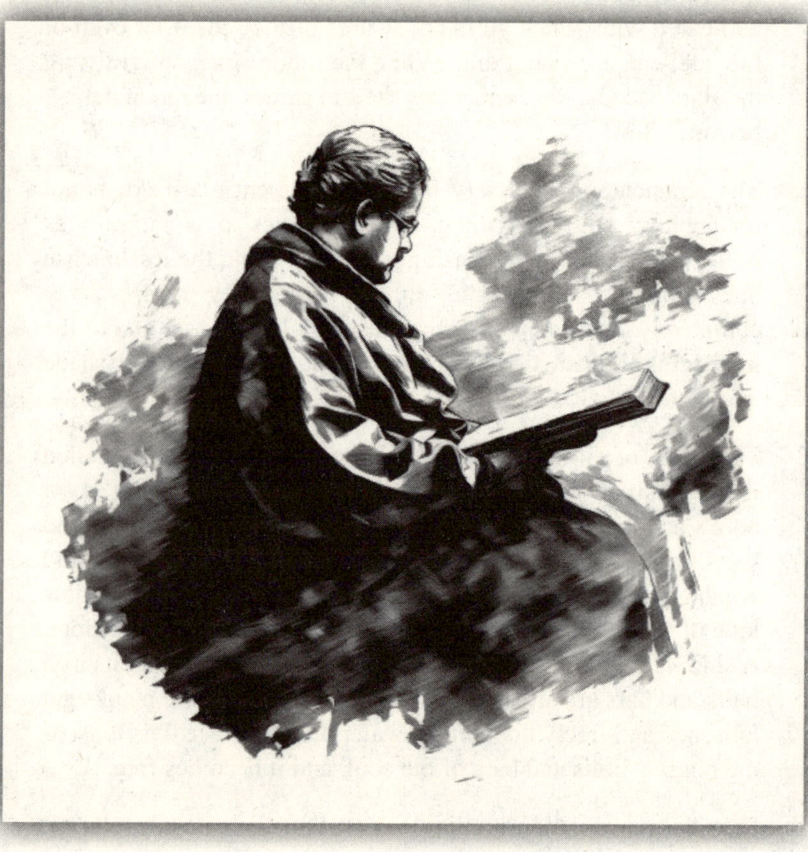

# The First Steps

The philosophers who wrote on Bhakti defined it as extreme love for God. Why a man should love God is the question to be solved; and until we understand that, we shall not be able to grasp the subject at all. There are two entirely different ideals of life. A man of any country who has any religion knows that he is a body and a spirit also. But there is a great deal of difference as to the goal of human life.

In Western countries, as a rule, people lay more stress on the body aspect of man; those philosophers who wrote on Bhakti in India laid stress on the spiritual side of man; and this difference seems to be typical of the Oriental and Occidental nations. It is so even in common language.

In England, when speaking of death it is said, a man gave up his ghost; in India, a man gave up his body. The one idea is that man is a body and has a soul; the other that man is a soul and has a body.

More intricate problems arise out of this. It naturally follows that the ideal which holds that man is a body and has a soul lays all the stress on the body. If you ask why man lives, you will be told it is to enjoy the senses, to enjoy possessions and wealth. He cannot dream of anything beyond even if he is told of it; his idea of a future life would be a continuation of this enjoyment.

He is very sorry that it cannot continue all the time here, but he has to depart; and he thinks that somehow or other he will go to some place where the same thing will be renewed. He will have the same enjoyments, the same senses, only heightened and strengthened. He wants to worship God, because God is the means to attain this end. The goal of his life is enjoyment of sense-objects, and he comes to know there is a Being who can give him a very long lease of these enjoyments, and that is why he worships God.

On the other hand the Indian idea is that God is the goal of life; there is nothing beyond God, and the sense-enjoyments are simply something through which we are passing now in the hope of getting better things. Not only so; it would be disastrous and terrible if man had nothing but sense-enjoyments. In our everyday life we find that the less the sense-enjoyments, the higher the life of the man.

Look at the dog when he eats. No man ever ate with the same satisfaction. Observe the pig giving grunts of satisfaction as he eats; it is his heaven, and if the greatest archangel came and looked on, the pig would not even notice him. His whole existence is in his eating. No man was ever born who could eat that way.

Think of the power of hearing in the lower animals, the power of seeing; all their senses are highly developed. Their enjoyment of the senses is extreme; they become simply mad with delight and pleasure. And the lower the man also, the more delight he finds in the senses. As he gets higher, the goal becomes reason and love. In proportion as these faculties develop, he loses the power of enjoying the senses.

For illustration's sake, if we take for granted that a certain amount of power is given to man, and that that can be spent either on the body, or the mind, or the spirit, then all the powers spent on any one of these leaves just so much less to be expended on the others. The ignorant or savage races have much stronger sensual faculties than the civilised races, and this is, in fact, one of the lessons we learn from history that as a nation becomes civilised the nerve organisation becomes finer, and they become physically weaker.

Civilise a savage race, and you will find the same thing; another barbarian race comes up and conquers it. It is nearly always the barbarian race that conquers. We see then that if we desire only to have sense-enjoyments all the time, we degrade ourselves to the brute state. A man does not know what he is asking for when he says, he wants to go to a place where his sense-enjoyments will be intensified; that he can only have by going down to the brutes.

So with men desiring a heaven full of sense-pleasures. They are like swine wallowing in the mire of the senses, unable to see anything beyond. This sense-enjoyment is what they want, and the loss of it is the loss of heaven to them. These can never be Bhaktas in the highest sense of the word; they can never be true lovers of God. At the same time, though this lower ideal be followed for a time, it will also in course of time change, each man will find that there is something higher, of which he did not know, and so this clinging to life and to things of the senses will gradually die away.

When I was a little boy at school, I had a fight with another schoolfellow about some sweetmeats, and he being the stronger boy snatched them from my hand. I remember the feeling I had; I thought that boy was the most wicked boy ever born, and that as soon as I grew strong enough I would punish him; there was no punishment sufficient for his wickedness. We have both grown up now, and we are fast friends.

This world is full of babies to whom eating and drinking, and all these little cakes are everything. They will dream of these cakes, and their idea of future life is where these cakes will be plentiful. Think of the American Indian who believes that his future life will be in a place which is a very good hunting ground. Each one of us has an idea of a heaven just as we want it to be; but in course of time, as we grow older and see higher things, we catch higher glimpses beyond.

But let us not dispense with our ideas of future life in the ordinary way of modern times, by not believing in anything — that is destruction. The agnostic who thus destroys everything is mistaken, the Bhakta sees higher. The agnostic does not want to go to heaven, because he has none; while the Bhakta does not want to go to heaven, because he thinks it is child's play. What he wants is God.

What can be a higher end than God? God Himself is the highest goal of man; see Him, enjoy Him. We can never conceive anything higher, because God is perfection. We cannot conceive of any higher enjoyment than that of love, but this word love has different meanings. It does not mean the ordinary selfish love of the world; it is blasphemy to call that love. The love for our children and our wives is mere animal love; that love which is perfectly unselfish is the only love, and that is of God.

It is a very difficult thing to attain to. We are passing through all these different loves — love of children, father, mother, and so forth. We slowly exercise the faculty of love; but in the majority of cases we never learn anything from it, we become bound to one step, to one person. In some cases men come out of this bondage. Men are ever running after wives and wealth and fame in this world; sometimes they are hit very hard on the head, and they find out what this world really is.

No one in this world can really love anything but God. Man finds out that human love is all hollow. Men cannot love though they talk of it. The wife says she loves her husband and kisses him; but as soon as he dies, the first thing she thinks about is the bank account, and what she shall do the next day. The husband loves the wife; but when she becomes sick and loses her beauty, or becomes haggard, or makes a mistake, he ceases to care for her. All the love of the world is hypocrisy and hollowness.

A finite subject cannot love, nor a finite object be loved. When the object of the love of a man is dying every moment, and his mind also is constantly changing as he grows, what eternal love can you expect to find in the world? There cannot be any real love but in God: why then all these loves? These are mere stages. There is a power behind impelling us forward, we do not know where to seek for the real object, but this love is sending us forward in search of it.

Again and again we find out our mistake. We grasp something, and find it slips through our fingers, and then we grasp something else. Thus on and on we go, till at last comes light; we come to God, the only One who loves. His love knows no change and is ever ready to take us in.

How long would any of you bear with me if I injured you? He in whose mind is no anger, hatred, or envy, who never loses his balance, dies, or is born, who is he but God?

But the path to God is long and difficult, and very few people attain Him. We are all babies struggling. Millions of people make a trade of religion. A few men in a century attain to that love of God, and the whole country becomes blessed and hallowed. When a son of God appears, a whole country becomes blessed. It is true that few such are born in any one century in the whole world, but all should strive to attain that love of God. Who knows but you or I may be the next to attain? Let us struggle therefore.

We say that a wife loves her husband. She thinks that her whole soul is absorbed in him: a baby comes and half of it goes out to the baby, or more. She herself will feel that the same love of husband does not exist now. So with the father. We always find that when more intense objects of love come to us, the previous love slowly vanishes.

Children at school think that some of their schoolfellows are the dearest beings that they have in life, or their fathers or mothers are so; then comes the husband or wife, and immediately the old feeling disappears, and the new love becomes uppermost. One star arises, another bigger one comes, and then a still bigger one, and at last the sun comes, and all the lesser lights vanish.

That sun is God. The stars are the smaller loves. When that Sun bursts upon him, a man becomes mad what Emerson calls "a God-intoxicated man". Man becomes transfigured into God, everything is merged in that one ocean of love. Ordinary love is mere animal attraction. Otherwise why is the distinction between the sexes? If one kneels before an image, it is dreadful idolatry; but if one kneels before husband or wife, it is quite permissible!

The world presents to us manifold stages of love. We have first to clear the ground. Upon our view of life the whole theory of love will rest. To think that this world is the aim and end of life is brutal and degenerating.

Any man who starts in life with that idea degenerates himself. He will never rise higher, he will never catch this glimpse from behind, he will always be a slave to the senses. He will struggle for the dollar that will get him a few cakes to eat. Better die than live that life. Slaves of this world, slaves of the senses, let us rouse ourselves; there is something higher than this sense-life.

Do you think that man, the Infinite Spirit was born to be a slave to his eyes, his nose, and his ears? There is an Infinite, Omniscient Spirit behind that can do everything, break every bond; and that Spirit we are, and we get that power through love. This is the ideal we must remember. We cannot, of course, get it in a day. We may fancy that we have it, but it is a fancy after all; it is a long, long way off. We must take man where he stands, and help him upwards. Man stands in materialism; you and I are materialists.

Our talking about God and Spirit is good; but it is simply the vogue in our society to talk thus: we have learnt it parrot-like and repeat it. So we have to take ourselves where we are as materialists, and must take the help of matter and go on slowly until we become real spiritualists, and feel ourselves spirits, understand the spirit, and find that this world which we call the infinite is but a gross external form of that world which is behind.

But something besides that is necessary. You read in the Sermon on the Mount, "Ask, and it shall be given (to) you; seek, and ye shall find; knock, and it shall be opened unto you."

The difficulty is, who seeks, who wants? We all say we know God. One man writes a book to disprove God, another to prove Him. One man thinks it his duty to prove Him all his life; another, to disprove Him, and he goes about to teach man there is no God.

What is the use of writing a book either to prove or disprove God? What does it matter to most people whether there is a God or not ? The majority of men work just like a machine with no thought of God and feeling no need of Him.

Then one day comes Death and says, "Come."

The man says, "Wait a little, I want a little more time. I want to see my son grow a little bigger." But Death says, "Come at once."

So it goes on. So goes poor John. What shall we say to poor John? He never found anything in which God was the highest; perhaps he was a pig in the past, and he is much better as a man. But there are some who get a little awakening. Some misery comes, someone whom we love most dies, that upon which we had bent our whole soul, that for which we had cheated the whole world and perhaps our own brother, that vanishes, and a blow comes to us.

Perhaps a voice comes in our soul and asks, "What after this?" Sometimes death comes without a blow, but such cases are few. Most of us, when anything slips through our fingers, say, "What next?" How we cling to the senses! You have heard of a drowning man clutching at a straw; a man will clutch at a straw first, and when it fails, he will say someone must help him. Still people must, as the English phrase goes, "sow their wild oats", before they can rise to higher things.

Bhakti is a religion. Religion is not for the many, that is impossible. A sort of knee-drill, standing up and sitting down, may be suited for the many; but religion is for the few. There are in every country only a few hundreds who can be, and will be religious. The others cannot be religious, because they will not be awakened, and they do not want to be.

The chief thing is to want God. We want everything except God, because our ordinary wants are supplied by the external world; it is only when our necessities have gone beyond the external world that we want a supply from the internal, from God.

So long as our needs are confined within the narrow limits of this physical universe, we cannot have any need for God; it is only when we have become satiated with everything here that we look beyond for a supply. It is only when the need is there that the demand will come. Have done with this child's play of the world as soon as you can, and then you will feel the necessity of something beyond the world, and the first step in religion will come.

There is a form of religion which is fashionable. My friend has much furniture in her parlour; it is the fashion to have a Japanese vase, so she must have one even if it costs a thousand dollars. In the same way she will have a little religion and join a church. Bhakti is not for such. That is not want.

Want is that without which we cannot live. We want breath, we want food, we want clothes; without them we cannot live. When a man loves a woman in this world, there are times when he feels that without her he cannot live, although that is a mistake. When a husband dies, the wife thinks she cannot live without him; but she lives all the same. This is the secret of necessity: it is that without which we cannot live; either it must come to us or we die.

When the time comes that we feel the same about God, or in other words, we want something beyond this world, something above all material forces, then we may become Bhaktas. What are our little lives when for a moment the cloud passes away, and we get one glimpse from beyond, and for that moment all these lower desires seem like a drop in the ocean? Then the soul grows, and feels the want of God, and must have Him.

The first step is: What do we want? Let us ask ourselves this question every day, do we want God? You may read all the books in the universe, but this love is not to be had by the power of speech, not by the highest intellect, not by the study of various sciences. He who desires God will get Love, unto him God gives Himself. Love is always mutual, reflective. You may hate me, and if I want to love you, you repulse me. But if I persist, in a month or a year you are bound to love me.

It is a wellknown psychological phenomenon. As the loving wife thinks of her departed husband, with the same love we must desire the Lord, and then we will find God, and all books and the various sciences would not be able to teach us anything. By reading books we become parrots; no one becomes learned by reading books. If a man reads but one word of love, he indeed becomes learned. So we want first to get that desire.

Let us ask ourselves each day, "Do we want Gods" When we begin to talk religion, and especially when we take a high position and begin to teach others, we must ask ourselves the same question. I find many times that I don't want God, I want bread more. I may go mad if I don't get a piece of bread; many ladies will go mad if they don't get a diamond pin, but they do not have the same desire for God; they do not know the only Reality that is in the universe.

There is a proverb in our language — If I want to be a hunter, I'll hunt the rhinoceros; if I want to be a robber, I'll rob the king's treasury. What is the use of robbing beggars or hunting ants? So if you want to love, love God. Who cares for these things of the world?

This world is utterly false; all the great teachers of the world found that out; there is no way out of it but through God. He is the goal of our life; all ideas that the world is the goal of life are pernicious. This world and this body have their own value, a secondary value, as a means to an end; but the world should not be the end.

Unfortunately, too often we make the world the end and God the means. We find people going to church and saying, "God, give me such and such; God, heal my disease." They want nice healthy bodies; and because they hear that someone will do this work for them, they go and pray to Him. It is better to be an atheist than to have such an idea of religion.

As I have told you, this Bhakti is the highest ideal; I don't know whether we shall reach it or not in millions of years to come, but we must make it our highest ideal, make our senses aim at the highest. If we cannot get to the end, we shall at least come nearer to it. We have slowly to work through the world and the senses to reach God.

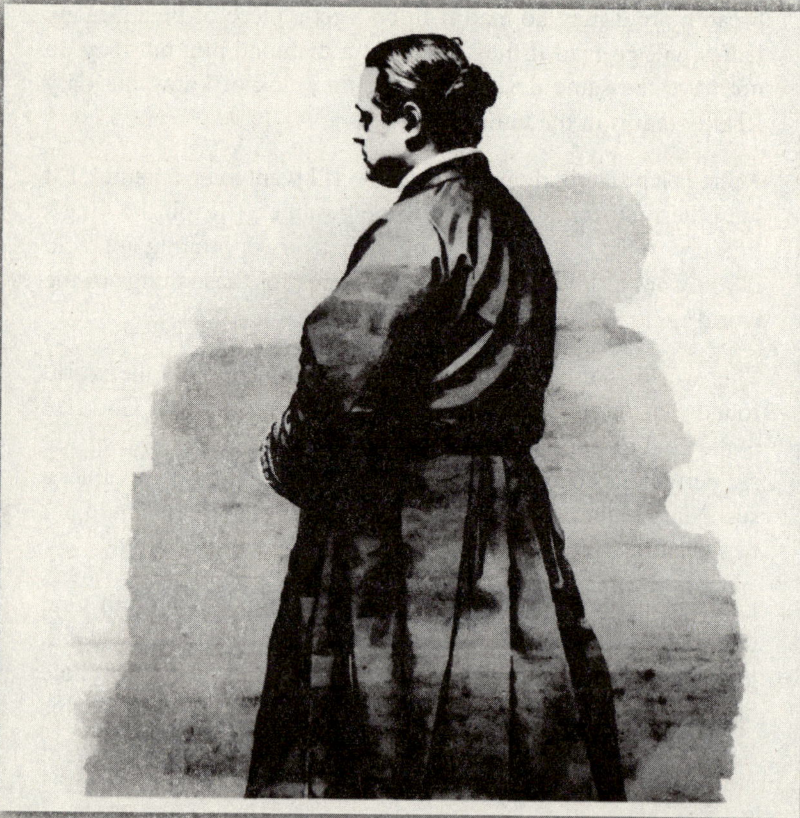

# The Need of Symbols

Bhakti is divided into two portions. One is called Vaidhi, formal or ceremonial; the other portion is called Mukhyâ, supreme. The word Bhakti covers all the ground between the lowest form of worship and the highest form of life. All the worship that you have seen in any country in the world, or in any religion, is regulated by love.

There is a good deal that is simple ceremony; there is also a good deal which, though not ceremony, is still not love, but a lower state. Yet these ceremonies are necessary. The external part of Bhakti is absolutely necessary to help the soul onward.

Man makes a great mistake when he thinks that he can at once jump to the highest state. If a baby thinks he is going to be an old man in a day, he is mistaken; and I hope you will always bear in mind this one ideal, that religion is neither in books, nor in intellectual consent, nor in reasoning. Reason, theories, documents, doctrines, books, religious ceremonies, are all helps to religion: religion itself consists in realisation .

We all say, "There is a God." Have you seen God? That is the question. You hear a man say, "There is God in heaven." You ask him if he has seen Him, and if he says he has, you would laugh at him and say he is a maniac. With most people religion is a sort of intellectual assent and goes no further than a document. I would not call it religion. It is better to be an atheist than to have that sort of religion. Religion does not depend on our intellectual assent or dissent.

You say there is a soul. Have you seen the soul? How is it we all have souls and do not see them? You have to answer the question and find out the way to see the soul. If not, it is useless to talk of religion. If any religion is true, it must be able to show us the soul and show us God and the truth in ourselves.

If you and I fight for all eternity about one of these doctrines or documents, we shall never come to any conclusion. People have been fighting for ages, and what is the outcome? Intellect cannot reach there at all. We have to go beyond the intellect; the proof of religion is in direct perception.

The proof of the existence of this wall is that we see it; if you sat down and argued about its existence or non-existence for ages, you could never come to any conclusion; but directly you see it, it is enough. If all the men in the world told you it did not exist, you would not believe them, because you know that the evidence of your own eyes is superior to that of all the doctrines and documents in the world.

To be religious, you have first to throw books overboard. The less you read of books, the better for you; do one thing at a time. It is a tendency in Western countries, in these modern times, to make a hotchpotch of the brain; all sorts of unassimilated ideas run riot in the brain and form a chaos without ever obtaining a chance to settle down and crystallise into a definite shape. In many cases it becomes a sort of disease, but this is not religion.

Then some want a sensation. Tell them about ghosts and people coming from the North Pole or any other remote place, with wings or in any other form, and that they are invisibly present and watching over them, and make them feel uncanny, then they are satisfied and go home; but within twenty-four hours they are ready for a fresh sensation. This is what some call religion.

This is the way to the lunatic asylum, and not to religion. The Lord is not to be reached by the weak, and all these weird things tend to weakness. Therefore go not near them; they only make people weak, bring disorder to the brain, weaken the mind, demoralise the soul, and a hopeless muddle is the result. You must bear in mind that religion does not consist in talk, or doctrines, or books, but in realisation; it is not learning, but being.

Everybody knows, "Do not steal", but what of it? That man has really known who has not stolen. Everybody knows, "Do not injure others", but of what value is it? Those who have not done so have realised it, they know it and have built their character on it. Religion is realising; and I will call you a worshipper of God when you have become able to realise the Idea. Before that it is the spelling of the weird, and no more. It is this power of realisation that makes religion. No amount of doctrines or philosophies or ethical books, that you may have stuffed into your brain, will matter much, only what you are and what you have realised.

So we have to realise religion, and this realisation of religion is a long process. When men hear of something very high and wonderful, they all think they will get that, and never stop for a moment to consider that they will have to work their way up to it; they all want to jump there. If it is the highest, we are for it. We never stop to consider whether we have the power, and the result is that we do not do anything. You cannot take a man with a pitchfork and push him up there; we all have to work up gradually. Therefore the first part of religion is Vaidhi Bhakti, the lower phase of worship.

What are these lower phases of worship? They are various. In order to attain to the state where we can realise, we must pass through the concrete — just as you see children learn through the concrete first — and gradually come to the abstract. If you tell a baby that five times two is ten, it will not understand; but if you bring ten things and show how five times two is ten, it will understand.

Religion is a long, slow process. We are all of us babies here; we may be old, and have studied all the books in the universe, but we are all spiritual babies. We have learnt the doctrines and dogmas, but realised nothing in our lives. We shall have to begin now in the concrete, through forms and words, prayers and ceremonies; and of these concrete forms there will be thousands; one form need not be for everybody.

Some may be helped by images, some may not. Some require an image outside, others one inside the brain. The man who puts it inside says, "I am a superior man. When it is inside it is all right; when it is outside, it is idolatry, I will fight it." When a man puts an image in the form of a church or a temple, he thinks it is holy; but when it is in a human form, he objects to it!

So there are various forms through which the mind will take this concrete exercise; and then, step by step, we shall come to the abstract understanding, abstract realisation. Again, the same form is not for everyone; there is one form that will suit you, and another will suit somebody else, and so on. All forms, though leading to the same goal, may not be for all of us.

Here is another mistake we generally make. My ideal does not suit you; and why should I force it on you? My fashion of building churches or reading hymns does not suit you; why should I force it on you? Go into the world and every fool will tell you that his form is the only right one, that every other form is diabolical, and he is the only chosen man ever born in the universe.

But in fact, all these forms are good and helpful. Just as there are certain varieties in human nature, so it is necessary that there should be an equal number of forms in religion; and the more there are, the better for the world. If there are twenty forms of religion in the world, it is very good; if there are four hundred, so much the better — there will be the more to choose from.

So we should rather be glad when the number of religions and religious ideas increase and multiply, because they will then include every man and help mankind more. Would to God that religions multiplied until every man had his own religion, quite separate from that of any other! This is the idea of the Bhakti-Yogi.

The final idea is that my religion cannot be yours, or yours mine. Although the goal and the aim are the same, yet each one has to take a different road, according to the tendencies of his mind; and although these roads are various, they must all be true, because they lead to the same goal. It cannot be that one is true and the rest not. The choosing of one's own road is called in the language of Bhakti, Ishta, the chosen way.

Then there are words. All of you have heard of the power of

words, how wonderful they are! Every book — the Bible, the Koran, and the Vedas — is full of the power of words. Certain words have wonderful power over mankind. Again, there are other forms, known as symbols. Symbols have great influence on the human mind.

But great symbols in religion were not created indefinitely. We find that they are the natural expressions of thought. We think symbolically. All our words are but symbols of the thought behind, and different people have come to use different symbols without knowing the reason why. It was all behind, and these symbols are associated with the thoughts; and as the thought brings the symbol outside, so the symbol, on the contrary, can bring the thought inside.

So one portion of Bhakti tells about these various subjects of symbols and words and prayers. Every religion has prayers, but one thing you must bear in mind — praying for health or wealth is not Bhakti, it is all Karma or meritorious action. Praying for any physical gain is simply Karma, such as a prayer for going to heaven and so forth.

One that wants to love God, to be a Bhakta, must discard all such prayers. He who wants to enter the realms of light must first give up this buying and selling this "shopkeeping" religion, and then enter the gates. It is not that you do not get what you pray for; you get everything, but such praying is a beggar's religion.

"Foolish indeed is he who, living on the banks of the Ganga, digs a little well for water. A fool indeed is the man who, coming to a mine of diamonds, seeks for glass beads."

This body will die some time, so what is the use of praying for its health again and again? What is there in health and wealth? The wealthiest man can use and enjoy only a little portion of his wealth. We can never get all the things of this world; and if not, who cares? This body will go, who cares for these things? If good things come, welcome; if they go away, let them go. Blessed are they when they come, and blessed are they when they go.

We are striving to come into the presence of the King of kings. We cannot get there in a beggar's dress. Even if we wanted to enter the presence of an emperor, should we be admitted? Certainly not. We should be driven out. This is the Emperor of emperors, and in these beggar's rags we cannot enter. Shopkeepers never have admission there; buying and selling have no place there.

As you read in the Bible, Jesus drove the buyers and sellers out of the Temple. Do not pray for little things. If you seek only bodily comforts, where is the difference between men and animals? Think yourselves a little higher than that.

So it goes without saying that the first task in becoming a Bhakta is to give up all desires of heaven and other things. The question is how to get rid of these desires. What makes men miserable? Because they are slaves, bound by laws, puppets in the hand of nature, tumbled about like playthings. We are continually taking care of this body that anything can knock down; and so we are living in a constant state of fear.

I have read that a deer has to run on the average sixty or seventy miles every day, because it is frightened. We ought to know that we are in a worse plight than the deer. The deer has some rest, but we have none. If the deer gets grass enough it is satisfied, but we are always multiplying our wants.

It is a morbid desire with us to multiply our wants. We have become so unhinged and unnatural that nothing natural will satisfy us. We are always grasping after morbid things, must have unnatural excitement — unnatural food, drink, surroundings, and life.

As to fear, what are our lives but bundles of fear? The deer has only one class of fear, such as that from tigers, wolves, etc. Man has the whole universe to fear.

How are we to free ourselves from this is the question. Utilitarians say, "Don't talk of God and hereafter; we don't know anything of these things, let us live happily in this world."

I would be the first to do so if we could, but the world will not allow us. As long as you are a slave of nature, how can you? The more you struggle, the more enveloped you become. You have been devising plans to make you happy, I do not know for how many years, but each year things seem to grow worse. Two hundred years ago in the old world people had few wants; but if their knowledge increased in arithmetical progression, their wants increased in geometrical progression.

We think that in salvation at least our desires will be fulfilled, so we desire to go to heaven. This eternal, unquenchable thirst! Always wanting something! When a man is a beggar, he wants money. When he has money, he wants other things, society; and after that, something else. Never at rest. How are we to quench this? If we get to heaven, it will only increase desire. If a poor man gets rich, it does not quench his desires, it is only like throwing butter on the fire, increasing its bright flames. Going to heaven means becoming intensely richer, and then desire comes more and more.

We read of many human things in heaven in the different Bibles of the world; they are not always very good there; and after all, this desire to go to heaven is a desire after enjoyment. This has to be given up. It is too little, too vulgar a thing for you to think of going to heaven. It is just the same as thinking, I will become a millionaire and lord it over people. There are many of these heavens, but through them you cannot gain the right to enter the gates of religion and love.

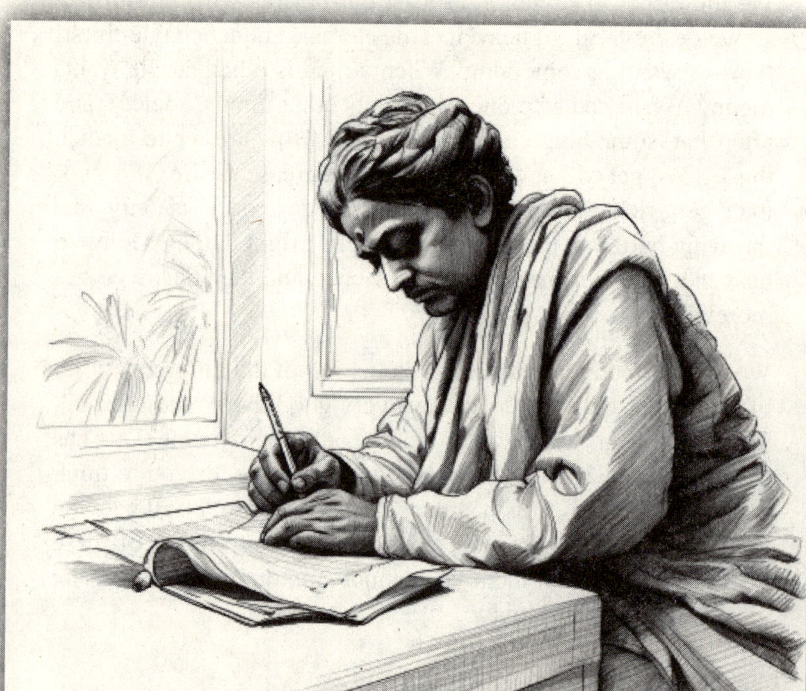

# Karma

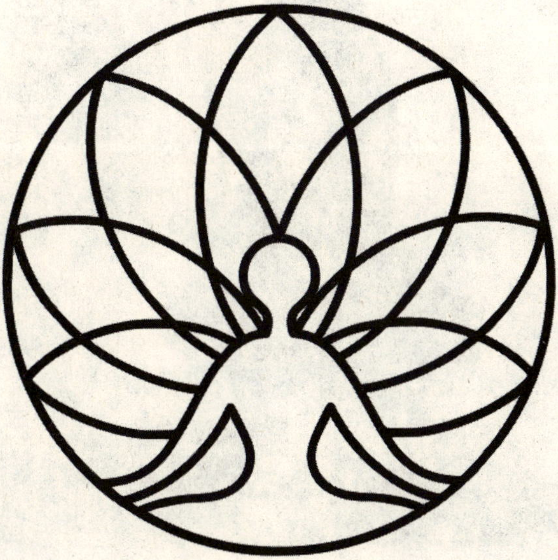

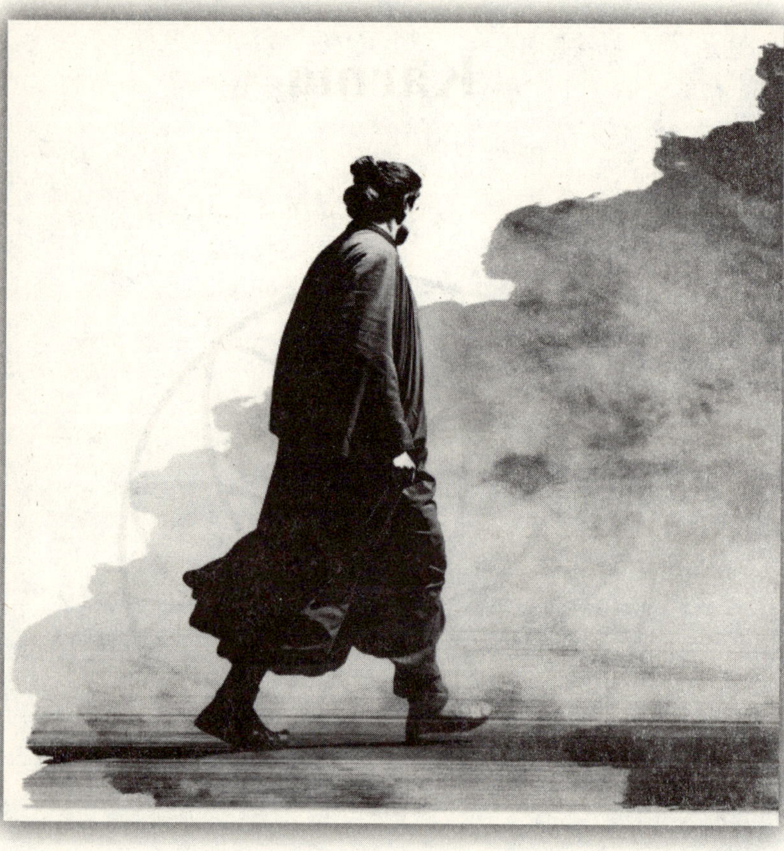

## The Theory of Karma

The theory of Karma is that we suffer for our good or bad deeds, and the whole scope of philosophy is to reach the glory of man. All the scriptures sing the glory of man, of the soul, and then, in the same breath, they preach Karma.

A good deed brings such a result, and a bad deed such another, but if the soul can be acted upon by a good or a bad deed, the soul amounts to nothing. Bad deeds put a bar to the manifestation of the nature of the Purusha; good deeds take the obstacles off, and the glory of the Purusha becomes manifest.

The Purusha itself is never changed. Whatever you do never destroys your own glory, your own nature, because the soul cannot be acted upon by anything, only a veil is spread before it, hiding its perfection.

With a view to exhausting their Karma quickly, Yogis create Kâya-vyuha, or groups of bodies, in which to work it out. For all these bodies they create minds from egoism. These are called "created minds", in contradistinction to their original minds.

Karma is the law of causation applied to conduct. According to this doctrine we must work forever, and the only way to get rid of pain is to do good works and thus to enjoy the good effects; and after living a life of good works, die and go to heaven and live forever in happiness. Even in heaven we could not be free from Karma, only it would be good Karma, not bad.

The philosophical portion denounces all work however good, and all pleasure, as loving and kissing wife, husband or children, as useless. According to this doctrine all good works and pleasures are nothing but foolishness and in their very nature impermanent. "All this must come to an end sometime, so end it now; it is vain." So says the philosophical portion of the Upanishads. It claims all the pain in the world is caused by ignorance, therefore the cure is knowledge.

This idea of one being held down fast by past Karma, or work, is all nonsense. No matter how dense one may be, or how bad, one ray of light will dissipate it all. A bale of cotton, however large, will be utterly destroyed by a spark. If a room has been dark for untold ages, a lamp will end it all. So with each soul, however benighted he may be, he is not absolutely bound down by his past Karma to work for ages to come. "One ray of Divine Light will free him, reveal to him his true nature."

Works are neither black nor white for the Yogis; for others they are threefold — black, white, and mixed.

When the Yogi has attained perfection, his actions, and the Karma produced by those actions, do not bind him, because he did not desire them. He just works on; he works to do good, and he does good, but does not care for the result, and it will not come to him. But, for ordinary men, who have not attained to the highest state, works are of three kinds, black (evil actions), white (good actions), and mixed.

From these threefold works are manifested in each state only those desires (which are) fitting to that state alone. (The others are held in abeyance for the time being.)

Suppose I have made the three kinds of Karma, good, bad, and mixed, and suppose I die and become a god in heaven. The desires in a god body are not the same as the desires in a human body; the god body neither eats nor drinks.

What becomes of my past unworked Karmas which produce as their effect the desire to eat and drink? Where would these Karmas go when I become a god?

The answer is that desires can only manifest themselves in proper environments. Only those desires will come out for which the environment is fitted; the rest will remain stored up.

In this life we have many godly desires, many human desires, many animal desires. If I take a god body, only the good desires will come up, because for them the environments are suitable. And if I take an animal body, only the animal desires will come up, and the good desires will wait.

What does this show? That by means of environment we can check these desires. Only that Karma which is suited to and fitted for the environments will come out. This shows that the power of environment is the great check to control even Karma itself.

Karma means work which will produce effect. When a man dies and becomes a Deva, he has only a period of pleasure, and during that time makes no fresh Karma; it is simply a reward for his past good Karma. When the good Karma is worked out, then the remaining Karma begins to take effect, and he comes down to earth. He becomes man again, and if he does very good works, and purifies himself, he goes to Brahmaloka and comes back no more.

The Lord can never be hoodwinked. The law of Karma can never be hoodwinked.

In the Vedas, there is no mention of hell. But our Purânas, the later books of our scriptures, thought that no religion could be complete, unless hells were attached to it. And so they invented all sorts of hells.

In some of these, men are sawed in half, and continually tortured, but do not die. They are continually feeling intense pain, but the books are merciful enough to say it is only for a period. Bad Karma is worked out in that state and then they come back on earth, and get another chance.

So this human form is the great chance. It is called the Karma-body, in which we decide our fate. We are running in a huge circle, and this is the point in the circle which determines the future. So this is considered the most important form that there is. Man is greater than the gods.

This earth is called the Karma-Bhumi, the sphere of Karma. Here alone man makes his good or bad Karma. When a man wants to go to heaven and does good works for that purpose, he becomes as good and does not as such store up any bad Karma. He just enjoys the effects of the good work he did on earth; and when this good Karma is exhausted, there come, upon him the resultant force of all the evil Karma he had previously stored up in life, and that brings him down again to this earth.

In the same way, those that become ghosts remain in that state, not giving rise to fresh Karma, but suffer the evil results of their past misdeeds, and later on remain for a time in an animal body without causing any fresh Karma. When that period is finished, they too become men again.

The states of reward and punishment due to good and bad Karmas are devoid of the force generating fresh Karmas; they have only to be enjoyed or suffered. If there is an extraordinarily good or an extraordinarily evil Karma, it bears fruit very quickly.

For instance, if a man has been doing many evil things all his life, but does one good act, the result of that good act will immediately appear. But when that result has been gone through, all the evil acts must produce their results also.

All men who do certain good and great acts, but the general tenor of whose lives has not been correct, will become gods; and after living for some time in god-bodies, enjoying the powers of gods, they will have again to become men; when the power of the good acts is thus finished, the old evil comes up to be worked out.

Those who do extraordinarily evil acts have to put on ghost and devil bodies, and when the effect of those evil actions is exhausted, the little good action which remains associated with them, makes them again become men. The way to Brahmaloka, from which there is no more fall or return, is called the Devayâna, i.e. the way to God; the way to heaven is known as Pitriyâna, i.e. the way to the fathers.

Man, therefore, according to the Vedanta philosophy, is the greatest being that is in the universe, and this world of work the best place in it, because only herein is the greatest and the best chance for him to become perfect. Angels or gods, whatever you may call them, have all to become men, if they want to become perfect. This is the great centre, the wonderful poise, and the wonderful opportunity — this human life.

Death overtakes everything which is complex. The soul is a single element, not composed of anything else, and therefore it cannot die. By its very nature the soul must be immortal. Body, mind, and soul turn upon the wheel of law — none can escape. No more can we transcend the law than can the stars, than can the sun — it is all a universe of law.

The law of Karma is that every action must be followed sooner or later by an effect. The Egyptian seed which was taken from the hand of a mummy after 5000 years and sprang into life when planted is the type of the never-ending influence of human acts. Action can never die without producing action.

Now, if our acts can only produce their appropriate effects on this plane of existence, it follows that we must all come back to round out the circle of causes and effects. This is the doctrine of reincarnation. We are the slaves of law, the slaves of conduct, the slaves of thirst, the slaves of desire, the slaves of a thousand things.

Only by escaping from life can we escape from slavery to freedom. God is the only one who is free. God and freedom are one and the same.

When we consider law in relation to man's mind and existence, it is at once obvious that there can be no such thing as free will and free existence. We know how animal nature is wholly regulated by law. The animal does not appear to exercise any free will. The same is true of man; human nature also is bound by law. The law governing functions of the human mind is called the law of Karma.

Nobody has ever seen anything produced out of nothing; if anything arises in the mind, that also must have been produced from something. When we speak of free will, we mean the will is not caused by anything. But that cannot be true, the will is caused; and since it is caused, it cannot be free — it is bound by law. That I am willing to talk to you and you come to listen to me, that is law. Everything that I do or think or feel, every part of my conduct or behaviour, my every movement — all is caused and therefore not free. This regulation of our life and mind — that is the law of Karma.

It is Karma that brings us together, and Karma separates.

Love everyone as your own self, because the whole universe is one. In injuring another, I am injuring myself; in loving another, I am loving myself. From this also springs that principle of Advaita morality which has been summed up in one word — self-abnegation.

The Advaitist says, this little personalised self is the cause of all my misery. This individualised self, which makes me different from all other beings, brings hatred and jealousy and misery, struggle and all other evils. And when this idea has been got rid of, all struggle will cease, all misery vanish.

So this is to be given up. We must always hold ourselves ready, even to give up our lives for the lowest beings. When a man has become ready even to give up his life for a little insect, he has reached the perfection which the Advaitist wants to attain; and at that moment when he has become thus ready, the veil of ignorance falls away from him, and he will feel his own nature.

Even in this life, he will feel that he is one with the universe. For a time, as it were, the whole of this phenomenal world will disappear for him, and he will realise what he is. But so long as the Karma of this body remains, he will have to live.

This state, when the veil has vanished and yet the body remains for some time, is what the Vedantists call the Jivanmukti, the living freedom. If a man is deluded by a mirage for some time, and one day the mirage disappears — if it comes back again the next day, or at some future time, he will not be deluded. Before the mirage first broke, the man could not distinguish between the reality and the deception.

But when it has once broken, as long as he has organs and eyes to work with, he will see the image, but will no more be deluded. That fine distinction between the actual world and the mirage he has caught, and the latter cannot delude him any more.

So when the Vedantist has realised his own nature, the whole world has vanished for him. It will come back again, but no more the same world of misery. The prison of misery has become changed into Sat, Chit, Ânanda — Existence Absolute, Knowledge Absolute, Bliss Absolute — and the attainment of this is the goal of the Advaita Philosophy.

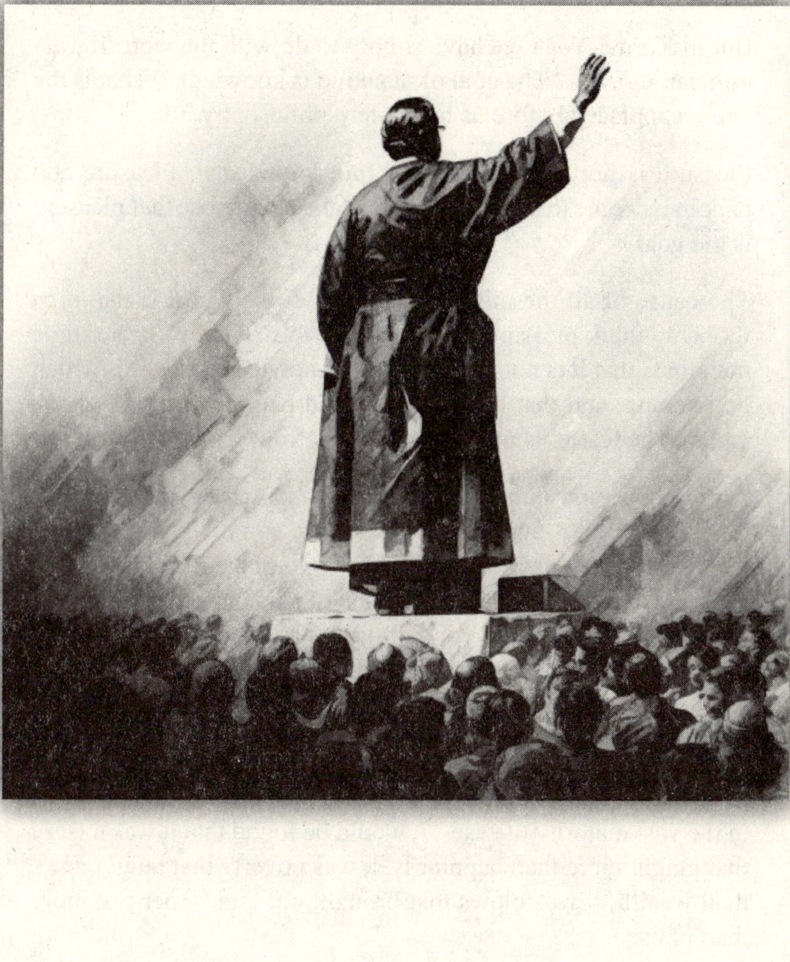

# Karma and Character

The word Karma is derived from the Sanskrit Kri, to do; all action is Karma. Technically, this word also means the effects of actions. In connection with metaphysics, it sometimes means the effects, of which our past actions were the causes.

But in Karma-Yoga we have simply to do with the word Karma as meaning work. The goal of mankind is knowledge. That is the one ideal placed before us by Eastern philosophy.

Pleasure is not the goal of man, but knowledge. Pleasure and happiness come to an end. It is a mistake to suppose that pleasure is the goal.

The cause of all the miseries we have in the world is that men foolishly think pleasure to be the ideal to strive for. After a time man finds that it is not happiness, but knowledge, towards which he is going, and that both pleasure and pain are great teachers, and that he learns as much from evil as from good.

As pleasure and pain pass before his soul they have upon it different pictures, and the result of these combined impressions is what is called man's "character". If you take the character of any man, it really is but the aggregate of tendencies, the sum total of the bent of his mind; you will find that misery and happiness are equal factors in the formation of that character.

Good and evil have an equal share in moulding character, and in some instances misery is a greater teacher than happiness. In studying the great characters the world has produced, I dare say, in the vast majority of cases, it would be found that it was misery that taught more than happiness, it was poverty that taught more than wealth, it was blows that brought out their inner fire more than praise.

Now this knowledge, again, is inherent in man. No knowledge comes from outside; it is all inside. What we say a man "knows", should, in strict psychological language, be what he "discovers" or "unveils"; what a man "learns" is really what he "discovers", by taking the cover off his own soul, which is a mine of infinite knowledge.

We say Newton discovered gravitation. Was it sitting anywhere in a corner waiting for him? It was in his own mind; the time came and he found it out. All knowledge that the world has ever received comes from the mind; the infinite library of the universe is in your own mind.

The external world is simply the suggestion, the occasion, which sets you to study your own mind, but the object of your study is always your own mind. The falling of an apple gave the suggestion to Newton, and he studied his own mind.

He rearranged all the previous links of thought in his mind and discovered a new link among them, which we call the law of gravitation. It was not in the apple nor in anything in the centre of the earth.

All knowledge, therefore, secular or spiritual, is in the human mind. In many cases it is not discovered, but remains covered, and when the covering is being slowly taken off, we say, "We are learning," and the advance of knowledge is made by the advance of this process of uncovering.

The man from whom this veil is being lifted is the more knowing man, the man upon whom it lies thick is ignorant, and the man from whom it has entirely gone is all-knowing, omniscient. There have been omniscient men, and, I believe, there will be yet; and that there will be myriads of them in the cycles to come.

Like fire in a piece of flint, knowledge exists in the mind; suggestion is the friction which brings it out. So with all our feelings and action — our tears and our smiles, our joys and our griefs, our weeping and our laughter, our curses and our blessings, our praises and our blames — every one of these we may find, if we calmly study our own selves, to have been brought out from within ourselves by so many blows. The result is what we are.

All these blows taken together are called Karma — work, action. Every mental and physical blow that is given to the soul, by which, as it were, fire is struck from it, and by which its own power and knowledge are discovered, is Karma, this word being used in its widest sense.

Thus we are all doing Karma all the time. I am talking to you: that is Karma. You are listening: that is Karma. We breathe: that is Karma. We walk: Karma. Everything we do, physical or mental, is Karma, and it leaves its marks on us.

There are certain works which are, as it were, the aggregate, the sum total, of a large number of smaller works. If we stand near the seashore and hear the waves dashing against the shingle, we think it is such a great noise, and yet we know that one wave is really composed of millions and millions of minute waves. Each one of these is making a noise, and yet we do not catch it; it is only when they become the big aggregate that we hear.

Similarly, every pulsation of the heart is work. Certain kinds of work we feel and they become tangible to us; they are, at the same time, the aggregate of a number of small works. If you really want to judge of the character of a man, look not at his great performances.

Every fool may become a hero at one time or another. Watch a man do his most common actions; those are indeed the things which will tell you the real character of a great man. Great occasions rouse even the lowest of human beings to some kind of greatness, but he alone is the really great man whose character is great always, the same wherever he be.

Karma in its effect on character is the most tremendous power that man has to deal with. Man is, as it were, a centre, and is attracting all the powers of the universe towards himself, and in this centre is fusing them all and again sending them off in a big current.

Such a centre is the real man — the almighty, the omniscient — and he draws the whole universe towards him. Good and bad, misery and happiness, all are running towards him and clinging round him; and out of them he fashions the mighty stream of tendency called character and throws it outwards. As he has the power of drawing in anything, so has he the power of throwing it out.

All the actions that we see in the world, all the movements in human society, all the works that we have around us, are simply the display of thought, the manifestation of the will of man. Machines or instruments, cities, ships, or men-of-war, all these are simply the manifestation of the will of man; and this will is caused by character, and character is manufactured by Karma.

As is Karma, so is the manifestation of the will. The men of mighty will the world has produced have all been tremendous workers — gigantic souls, with wills powerful enough to overturn worlds, wills they got by persistent work, through ages, and ages. Such a gigantic will as that of a Buddha or a Jesus could not be obtained in one life, for we know who their fathers were.

It is not known that their fathers ever spoke a word for the good of mankind. Millions and millions of carpenters like Joseph had gone; millions are still living. Millions and millions of petty kings like Buddha's father had been in the world.

If it was only a case of hereditary transmission, how do you account for this petty prince, who was not, perhaps, obeyed by his own servants, producing this son, whom half a world worships? How do you explain the gulf between the carpenter and his son, whom millions of human beings worship as God? It cannot be solved by the theory of heredity.

The gigantic will which Buddha and Jesus threw over the world, whence did it come? Whence came this accumulation of power? It must have been there through ages and ages, continually growing bigger and bigger, until it burst on society in a Buddha or a Jesus, even rolling down to the present day.

All this is determined by Karma, work. No one can get anything unless he earns it. This is an eternal law. We may sometimes think it is not so, but in the long run we become convinced of it.

A man may struggle all his life for riches; he may cheat thousands, but he finds at last that he did not deserve to become rich, and his life becomes a trouble and a nuisance to him. We may go on accumulating things for our physical enjoyment, but only what we earn is really ours.

A fool may buy all the books in the world, and they will be in his library; but he will be able to read only those that he deserves to; and this deserving is produced by Karma. Our Karma determines what we deserve and what we can assimilate. We are responsible for what we are; and whatever we wish ourselves to be, we have the power to make ourselves.

If what we are now has been the result of our own past actions, it certainly follows that whatever we wish to be in future can be produced by our present actions; so we have to know how to act.

You will say, "What is the use of learning how to work? Everyone works in some way or other in this world."

But there is such a thing as frittering away our energies. With regard to Karma-Yoga, the Gita says that it is doing work with cleverness and as a science; by knowing how to work, one can obtain the greatest results. You must remember that all work is simply to bring out the power of the mind which is already there, to wake up the soul. The power is inside every man, so is knowing; the different works are like blows to bring them out, to cause these giants to wake up.

Man works with various motives. There cannot be work without motive. Some people want to get fame, and they work for fame. Others want money, and they work for money. Others want to have power, and they work for power.

Others want to get to heaven, and they work for the same. Others want to leave a name when they die, as they do in China, where no man gets a title until he is dead; and that is a better way, after all, than with us.

When a man does something very good there, they give a title of nobility to his father, who is dead, or to his grandfather. Some people work for that.

Some of the followers of certain Mohammedan sects work all their lives to have a big tomb built for them when they die. I know sects among whom, as soon as a child is born, a tomb is prepared for it; that is among them the most important work a man has to do, and the bigger and the finer the tomb, the better off the man is supposed to be.

Others work as a penance; do all sorts of wicked things, then erect a temple, or give something to the priests to buy them off and obtain from them a passport to heaven. They think that this kind of beneficence will clear them and they will go scot-free in spite of their sinfulness. Such are some of the various motives for work.

Work for work's sake. There are some who are really the salt of the earth in every country and who work for work's sake, who do not care for name, or fame, or even to go to heaven. They work just because good will come of it.

There are others who do good to the poor and help mankind from still higher motives, because they believe in doing good and love good. The motive for name and fame seldom brings immediate results, as a rule; they come to us when we are old and have almost done with life.

If a man works without any selfish motive in view, does he not gain anything? Yes, he gains the highest. Unselfishness is more paying, only people have not the patience to practice it. It is more paying from the point of view of health also. Love, truth, and unselfishness are not merely moral figures of speech, but they form our highest ideal, because in them lies such a manifestation of power.

In the first place, a man who can work for five days, or even for five minutes, without any selfish motive whatever, without thinking of future, of heaven, of punishment, or anything of the kind, has in him the capacity to become a powerful moral giant. It is hard to do it, but in the heart of our hearts we know its value, and the good it brings. It is the greatest manifestation of power — this tremendous restraint; self-restraint is a manifestation of greater power than all outgoing action.

A carriage with four horses may rush down a hill unrestrained, or the coachman may curb the horses. Which is the greater manifestation of power, to let them go or to hold them? A cannonball flying through the air goes a long distance and falls.

Another is cut short in its flight by striking against a wall, and the impact generates intense heat. All outgoing energy following a selfish motive is frittered away; it will not cause power to return to you; but if restrained, it will result in development of power.

This self-control will tend to produce a mighty will, a character which makes a Christ or a Buddha. Foolish men do not know this secret; they nevertheless want to rule mankind. Even a fool may rule the whole world if he works and waits. Let him wait a few years, restrain that foolish idea of governing; and when that idea is wholly gone, he will be a power in the world.

The majority of us cannot see beyond a few years, just as some animals cannot see beyond a few steps. Just a little narrow circle — that is our world. We have not the patience to look beyond, and thus become immoral and wicked. This is our weakness, our powerlessness.

Even the lowest forms of work are not to be despised. Let the man, who knows no better, work for selfish ends, for name and fame; but everyone should always try to get towards higher and higher motives and to understand them. "To work we have the right, but not to the fruits thereof."

Leave the fruits alone. Why care for results? If you wish to help a man, never think what that man's attitude should be towards you. If you want to do a great or a good work, do not trouble to think what the result will be.

There arises a difficult question in this ideal of work. Intense activity is necessary; we must always work. We cannot live a minute without work.

What then becomes of rest? Here is one side of the life-struggle — work, in which we are whirled rapidly round. And here is the other — that of calm, retiring renunciation: everything is peaceful around, there is very little of noise and show, only nature with her animals and flowers and mountains.

Neither of them is a perfect picture. A man used to solitude, if brought in contact with the surging whirlpool of the world, will be crushed by it; just as the fish that lives in the deep sea water, as soon as it is brought to the surface, breaks into pieces, deprived of the weight of water on it that had kept it together.

Can a man who has been used to the turmoil and the rush of life live at ease if he comes to a quiet place? He suffers and perchance may lose his mind.

The ideal man is he who, in the midst of the greatest silence and solitude, finds the intensest activity, and in the midst of the intensest activity finds the silence and solitude of the desert. He has learnt the secret of restraint, he has controlled himself. He goes through the streets of a big city with all its traffic, and his mind is as calm as if he were in a cave, where not a sound could reach him; and he is intensely working all the time. That is the ideal of Karma-Yoga, and if you have attained to that you have really learnt the secret of work.

But we have to begin from the beginning, to take up the works as they come to us and slowly make ourselves more unselfish every day. We must do the work and find out the motive power that prompts us; and, almost without exception, in the first years, we shall find that our motives are always selfish; but gradually this selfishness will melt by persistence, till at last will come the time when we shall be able to do really unselfish work.

We may all hope that some day or other, as we struggle through the paths of life, there will come a time when we shall become perfectly unselfish; and the moment we attain to that, all our powers will be concentrated, and the knowledge which is ours will be manifest.

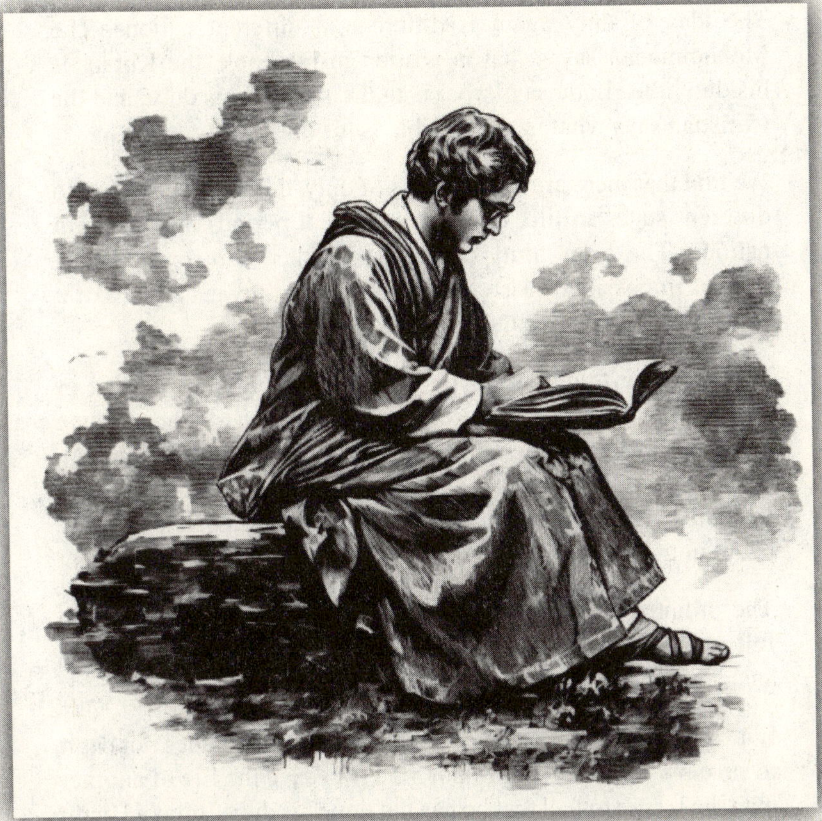

# What Is Duty?

It is necessary in the study of Karma-Yoga to know what duty is. If I have to do something I must first know that it is my duty, and then I can do it.

The idea of duty again is different in different nations. The Mohammedan says what is written in his book, the Koran, is his duty; the Hindu says what is in the Vedas is his duty; and the Christian says what is in the Bible is his duty.

We find that there are varied ideas of duty, differing according to different states in life, different historical periods and different nations. The term "duty", like every other universal abstract term, is impossible clearly to define; we can only get an idea of it by knowing its practical operations and results.

When certain things occur before us, we have all a natural or trained impulse to act in a certain manner towards them; when this impulse comes, the mind begins to think about the situation. Sometimes it thinks that it is good to act in a particular manner under the given conditions; at other times it thinks that it is wrong to act in the same manner even in the very same circumstances.

The ordinary idea of duty everywhere is that every good man follows the dictates of his conscience. But what is it that makes an act a duty?

If a Christian finds a piece of beef before him and does not eat it to save his own life, or will not give it to save the life of another man, he is sure to feel that he has not done his duty. But if a Hindu dares to eat that piece of beef or to give it to another Hindu, he is equally sure to feel that he too has not done his duty; the Hindu's training and education make him feel that way.

In the last century there were notorious bands of robbers in India called thugs; they thought it their duty to kill any man they could and take away his money; the larger the number of men they killed, the better they thought they were. Ordinarily if a man goes out into the street and shoots down another man, he is apt to feel sorry for it, thinking that he has done wrong. But if the very same man, as a soldier in his regiment, kills not one but twenty, he is certain to feel glad and think that he has done his duty remarkably well.

Therefore we see that it is not the thing done that defines a duty. To give an objective definition of duty is thus entirely impossible. Yet there is duty from the subjective side. Any action that makes us go Godward is a good action, and is our duty; any action that makes us go downward is evil, and is not our duty.

From the subjective standpoint we may see that certain acts have a tendency to exalt and ennoble us, while certain other acts have a tendency to degrade and to brutalise us. But it is not possible to make out with certainty which acts have which kind of tendency in relation to all persons, of all sorts and conditions.

There is, however, only one idea of duty which has been universally accepted by all mankind, of all ages and sects and countries, and that has been summed up in a Sanskrit aphorism thus: "Do not injure any being; not injuring any being is virtue, injuring any being is sin."

The Bhagavad-Gita frequently alludes to duties dependent upon birth and position in life. Birth and position in life and in society largely determine the mental and moral attitude of individuals towards the various activities of life. It is therefore our duty to do that work which will exalt and ennoble us in accordance with the ideals and activities of the society in which we are born.

But it must be particularly remembered that the same ideals and activities do not prevail in all societies and countries; our ignorance of this is the main cause of much of the hatred of one nation towards another. An American thinks that whatever an American does in accordance with the custom of his country is the best thing to do, and that whoever does not follow his custom must be a very wicked man. A Hindu thinks that his customs are the only right ones and are the best in the world, and that whosoever does not obey them must be the most wicked man living.

This is quite a natural mistake which all of us are apt to make. But it is very harmful; it is the cause of half the uncharitableness found in the world.

When I came to this country and was going through the Chicago Fair, a man from behind pulled at my turban. I looked back and saw that he was a very gentlemanly-looking man, neatly dressed. I spoke to him; and when he found that I knew English, he became very much abashed.

On another occasion in the same Fair another man gave me a push. When I asked him the reason, he also was ashamed and stammered out an apology saying, "Why do you dress that way?"

The sympathies of these men were limited within the range of their own language and their own fashion of dress. Much of the oppression of powerful nations on weaker ones is caused by this prejudice. It dries up their fellow feeling for fellow men. That very man who asked me why I did not dress as he did and wanted to ill-treat me because of my dress may have been a very good man, a good father, and a good citizen; but the kindliness of his nature died out as soon as he saw a man in a different dress.

Strangers are exploited in all countries, because they do not know how to defend themselves; thus they carry home false impressions of the peoples they have seen. Sailors, soldiers, and traders behave in foreign lands in very queer ways, although they would not dream of doing so in their own country; perhaps this is why the Chinese call Europeans and Americans "foreign devils". They could not have done this if they had met the good, the kindly sides of Western life.

Therefore the one point we ought to remember is that we should always try to see the duty of others through their own eyes, and never judge the customs of other peoples by our own standard. I am not the standard of the universe. I have to accommodate myself to the world, and not the world to me.

So we see that environments change the nature of our duties, and doing the duty which is ours at any particular time is the best thing we can do in this world. Let us do that duty which is ours by birth; and when we have done that, let us do the duty which is ours by our position in life and in society.

There is, however, one great danger in human nature, viz that man never examines himself. He thinks he is quite as fit to be on the throne as the king. Even if he is, he must first show that he has done the duty of his own position; and then higher duties will come to him.

When we begin to work earnestly in the world, nature gives us blows right and left and soon enables us to find out our position. No man can long occupy satisfactorily a position for which he is not fit. There is no use in grumbling against nature's adjustment. He who does the lower work is not therefore a lower man. No man is to be judged by the mere nature of his duties, but all should be judged by the manner and the spirit in which they perform them.

Later on we shall find that even this idea of duty undergoes change, and that the greatest work is done only when there is no selfish motive to prompt it. Yet it is work through the sense of duty that leads us to work without any idea of duty; when work will become worship — nay, something higher — then will work be done for its own sake.

We shall find that the philosophy of duty, whether it be in the form of ethics or of love, is the same as in every other Yoga — the object being the attenuating of the lower self, so that the real higher Self may shine forth — the lessening of the frittering away of energies on the lower plane of existence, so that the soul may manifest itself on the higher ones.

This is accomplished by the continuous denial of low desires, which duty rigorously requires. The whole organisation of society has thus been developed, consciously or unconsciously, in the realms of action and experience, where, by limiting selfishness, we open the way to an unlimited expansion of the real nature of man.

Duty is seldom sweet. It is only when love greases its wheels that it runs smoothly; it is a continuous friction otherwise. How else could parents do their duties to their children, husbands to their wives, and vice versa? Do we not meet with cases of friction every day in our lives? Duty is sweet only through love, and love shines in freedom alone.

Yet is it freedom to be a slave to the senses, to anger, to jealousies and a hundred other petty things that must occur every day in human life? In all these little roughnesses that we meet with in life, the highest expression of freedom is to forbear.

Women, slaves to their own irritable, jealous tempers, are apt to blame their husbands, and assert their own "freedom", as they think, not knowing that thereby they only prove that they are slaves. So it is with husbands who eternally find fault with their wives.

Chastity is the first virtue in man or woman, and the man who, however he may have strayed away, cannot be brought to the right path by a gentle and loving and chaste wife is indeed very rare. The world is not yet as bad as that.

We hear much about brutal husbands all over the world and about the impurity of men, but is it not true that there are quite as many brutal and impure women as men? If all women were as good and pure as their own constant assertions would lead one to believe, I am perfectly satisfied that there would not be one impure man in the world.

What brutality is there which purity and chastity cannot conquer? A good, chaste wife, who thinks of every other man except her own husband as her child and has the attitude of a mother towards all men, will grow so great in the power of her purity that there cannot be a single man, however brutal, who will not breathe an atmosphere of holiness in her presence.

Similarly, every husband must look upon all women, except his own wife, in the light of his own mother or daughter or sister. That man, again, who wants to be a teacher of religion must look upon every woman as his mother, and always behave towards her as such.

The position of the mother is the highest in the world, as it is the one place in which to learn and exercise the greatest unselfishness. The love of God is the only love that is higher than a mother's love; all others are lower.

It is the duty of the mother to think of her children first and then of herself. But, instead of that, if the parents are always thinking of themselves first, the result is that the relation between parents and children becomes the same as that between birds and their offspring which, as soon as they are fledged, do not recognise any parents.

Blessed, indeed, is the man who is able to look upon woman as the representative of the motherhood of God. Blessed, indeed, is the woman to whom man represents the fatherhood of God. Blessed are the children who look upon their parents as Divinity manifested on earth.

The only way to rise is by doing the duty next to us, and thus gathering strength go on until we reach the highest state. A young Sannyâsin went to a forest; there he meditated, worshipped, and practiced Yoga for a long time.

After years of hard work and practice, he was one day sitting under a tree, when some dry leaves fell upon his head. He looked up and saw a crow and a crane fighting on the top of the tree, which made him very angry.

He said, "What! Dare you throw these dry leaves upon my head!"

As with these words he angrily glanced at them, a flash of fire went out of his head — such was the Yogi's power — and burnt the birds to ashes. He was very glad, almost overjoyed at this development of power — he could burn the crow and the crane by a look.

After a time he had to go to the town to beg his bread. He went, stood at a door, and said, "Mother, give me food."

A voice came from inside the house, "Wait a little, my son."

The young man thought, "You wretched woman, how dare you make me wait! You do not know my power yet."

While he was thinking thus the voice came again: "Boy, don't be thinking too much of yourself. Here is neither crow nor crane."

He was astonished; still he had to wait. At last the woman came, and he fell at her feet and said, "Mother, how did you know that?"

She said, "My boy, I do not know your Yoga or your practices. I am a common everyday woman. I made you wait because my husband is ill, and I was nursing him. All my life I have struggled to do my duty. When I was unmarried, I did my duty to my parents; now that I am married, I do my duty to my husband; that is all the Yoga I practice. But by doing my duty I have become illumined; thus I could read your thoughts and know what you had done in the forest. If you want to know something higher than this, go to the market of such and such a town where you will find a Vyâdha (The lowest class of people in India who used to live as hunters and butchers.) who will tell you something that you will be very glad to learn."

The Sannyasin thought, "Why should I go to that town and to a Vyadha?"

But after what he had seen, his mind opened a little, so he went. When he came near the town, he found the market and there saw, at a distance, a big fat Vyadha cutting meat with big knives, talking and bargaining with different people.

The young man said, "Lord help me! Is this the man from whom I am going to learn? He is the incarnation of a demon, if he is anything."

In the meantime this man looked up and said, "O Swami, did that lady send you here? Take a seat until I have done my business."

The Sannyasin thought, "What comes to me here?"

He took his seat; the man went on with his work, and after he had finished he took his money and said to the Sannyasin, "Come sir, come to my home."

On reaching home the Vyadha gave him a seat, saying, "Wait here," and went into the house. He then washed his old father and mother, fed them, and did all he could to please them, after which he came to the Sannyasin and said, "Now, sir, you have come here to see me; what can I do for you?"

The Sannyasin asked him a few questions about soul and about God, and the Vyadha gave him a lecture which forms a part of the Mahâbhârata, called the Vyâdha-Gitâ. It contains one of the highest flights of the Vedanta.

When the Vyadha finished his teaching, the Sannyasin felt astonished. He said, "Why are you in that body? With such knowledge as yours why are you in a Vyadha's body, and doing such filthy, ugly work?"

"My son," replied the Vyadha, "no duty is ugly, no duty is impure. My birth placed me in these circumstances and environments. In my boyhood I learnt the trade; I am unattached, and I try to do my duty well. I try to do my duty as a householder, and I try to do all I can to make my father and mother happy. I neither know your Yoga, nor have I become a Sannyasin, nor did I go out of the world into a forest; nevertheless, all that you have heard and seen has come to me through the unattached doing of the duty which belongs to my position."

There is a sage in India, a great Yogi, one of the most wonderful men I have ever seen in my life. He is a peculiar man, he will not teach any one; if you ask him a question he will not answer. It is too much for him to take up the position of a teacher, he will not do it. If you ask a question, and wait for some days, in the course of conversation he will bring up the subject, and wonderful light will he throw on it.

He told me once the secret of work, "Let the end and the means be joined into one." When you are doing any work, do not think of anything beyond. Do it as worship, as the highest worship, and devote your whole life to it for the time being.

Thus, in the story, the Vyadha and the woman did their duty with cheerfulness and whole-heartedness; and the result was that they became illuminated, clearly showing that the right performance of the duties of any station in life, without attachment to results, leads us to the highest realisation of the perfection of the soul.

It is the worker who is attached to results that grumbles about the nature of the duty which has fallen to his lot. To the unattached worker all duties are equally good, and form efficient instruments with which selfishness and sensuality may be killed, and the freedom of the soul secured.

We are all apt to think too highly of ourselves. Our duties are determined by our desires to a much larger extent than we are willing to grant. Competition rouses envy, and it kills the kindliness of the heart. To the grumbler all duties are distasteful; nothing will ever satisfy him, and his whole life is doomed to prove a failure.

Let us work on, doing as we go whatever happens to be our duty, and being ever ready to put our shoulders to the wheel. Then surely shall we see the Light!

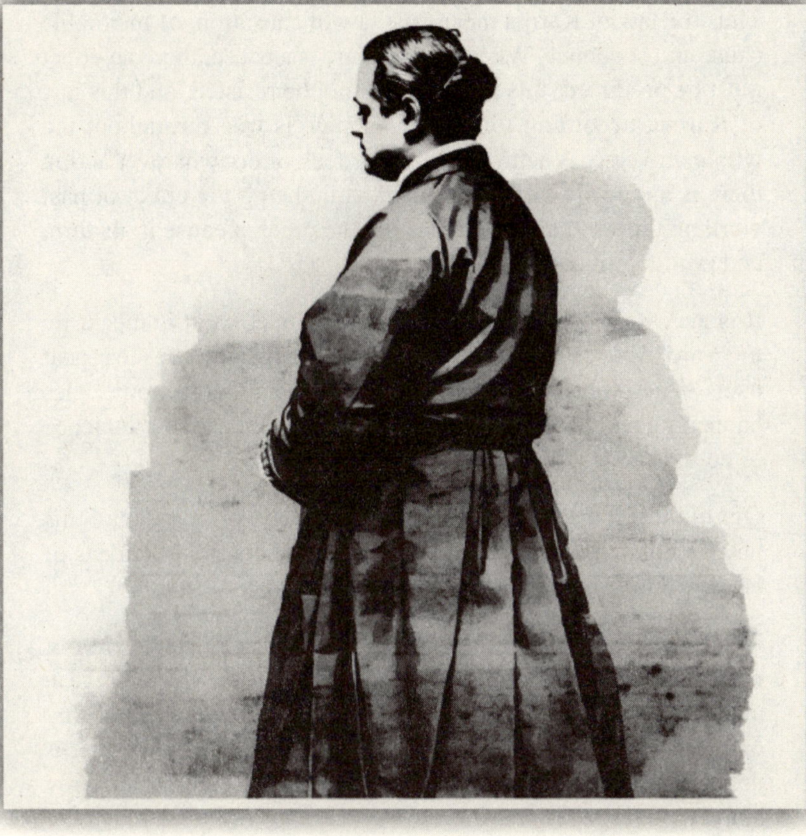

# Freedom

In addition to meaning work, we have stated that psychologically the word Karma also implies causation. Any work, any action, any thought that produces an effect is called a Karma.

Thus the law of Karma means the law of causation, of inevitable cause and sequence. Wheresoever there is a cause, there an effect must be produced; this necessity cannot be resisted, and this law of Karma, according to our philosophy, is true throughout the whole universe. Whatever we see, or feel, or do, whatever action there is anywhere in the universe, while being the effect of past work on the one hand, becomes, on the other, a cause in its turn, and produces its own effect.

It is necessary, together with this, to consider what is meant by the word "law". By law is meant the tendency of a series to repeat itself. When we see one event followed by another, or sometimes happening simultaneously with another, we expect this sequence or co-existence to recur.

Our old logicians and philosophers of the Nyâyâ school call this law by the name of Vyâpti. According to them, all our ideas of law are due to association.

A series of phenomena becomes associated with things in our mind in a sort of invariable order, so that whatever we perceive at any time is immediately referred to other facts in the mind. Any one idea or, according to our psychology, any one wave that is produced in the mind-stuff, Chitta, must always give rise to many similar waves.

This is the psychological idea of association, and causation is only an aspect of this grand pervasive principle of association. This pervasiveness of association is what is, in Sanskrit, called Vyâpti.

In the external world the idea of law is the same as in the internal

— the expectation that a particular phenomenon will be followed by another, and that the series will repeat itself. Really speaking, therefore, law does not exist in nature. Practically it is an error to say that gravitation exists in the earth, or that there is any law existing objectively anywhere in nature.

Law is the method, the manner in which our mind grasps a series of phenomena; it is all in the mind. Certain phenomena, happening one after another or together, and followed by the conviction of the regularity of their recurrence — thus enabling our minds to grasp the method of the whole series — constitute what we call law.

The next question for consideration is what we mean by law being universal. Our universe is that portion of existence which is characterized by what the Sanskrit psychologists call Desha-kâla-nimitta, or what is known to European psychology as space, time, and causation. This universe is only a part of infinite existence, thrown into a peculiar mould, composed of space, time, and causation.

It necessarily follows that law is possible only within this conditioned universe; beyond it there cannot be any law. When we speak of the universe, we only mean that portion of existence which is limited by our mind — the universe of the senses, which we can see, feel, touch, hear, think of, imagine. This alone is under law; but beyond it existence cannot be subject to law, because causation does not extend beyond the world of our minds.

Anything beyond the range of our mind and our senses is not bound by the law of causation, as there is no mental association of things in the region beyond the senses, and no causation without association of ideas. It is only when "being" or existence gets moulded into name and form that it obeys the law of causation, and is said to be under law; because all law has its essence in causation.

Therefore we see at once that there cannot be any such thing as free will; the very words are a contradiction, because will is what we know, and everything that we know is within our universe, and everything within our universe is moulded by the conditions of space, time, and causation. Everything that we know, or can possibly know, must be subject to causation, and that which obeys the law of causation cannot be free. It is acted upon by other agents, and becomes a cause in its turn.

But that which has become converted into the will, which was not the will before, but which, when it fell into this mould of space, time, and causation, became converted into the human will, is free; and when this will gets out of this mould of space, time, and causation, it will be free again. From freedom it comes, and becomes moulded into this bondage, and it gets out and goes back to freedom again.

The question has been raised as to from whom this universe comes, in whom it rests, and to whom it goes; and the answer has been given that from freedom it comes, in bondage it rests, and goes back into that freedom again. So, when we speak of man as no other than that infinite being which is manifesting itself, we mean that only one very small part thereof is man; this body and this mind which we see are only one part of the whole, only one spot of the infinite being.

This whole universe is only one speck of the infinite being; and all our laws, our bondages, our joys and our sorrows, our happinesses and our expectations, are only within this small universe; all our progression and digression are within its small compass.

So you see how childish it is to expect a continuation of this universe — the creation of our minds — and to expect to go to heaven, which after all must mean only a repetition of this world that we know. You see at once that it is an impossible and childish desire to make the whole of infinite existence conform to the limited and conditioned existence which we know.

When a man says that he will have again and again this same thing which he is hating now, or, as I sometimes put it, when he asks for a comfortable religion, you may know that he has become so degenerate that he cannot think of anything higher than what he is now. He is just his little present surroundings and nothing more.

He has forgotten his infinite nature, and his whole idea is confined to these little joys, and sorrows, and heart-jealousies of the moment. He thinks that this finite thing is the infinite; and not only so, he will not let this foolishness go.

He clings on desperately unto Trishnâ, and the thirst after life, what the Buddhists call Tanhâ and Tissâ. There may be millions of kinds of happiness, and beings, and laws, and progress, and causation, all acting outside the little universe that we know; and, after all, the whole of this comprises but one section of our infinite nature.

To acquire freedom we have to get beyond the limitations of this universe; it cannot be found here. Perfect equilibrium, or what the Christians call the peace that passeth all understanding, cannot be had in this universe, nor in heaven, nor in any place where our mind and thoughts can go, where the senses can feel, or which the imagination can conceive.

No such place can give us that freedom, because all such places would be within our universe, and it is limited by space, time, and causation. There may be places that are more ethereal than this earth of ours, where enjoyments may be keener, but even those places must be in the universe and, therefore, in bondage to law; so we have to go beyond, and real religion begins where this little universe ends.

These little joys, and sorrows, and knowledge of things end there, and the reality begins. Until we give up the thirst after life, the strong attachment to this our transient conditioned existence we have no hope of catching even a glimpse of that infinite freedom beyond.

It stands to reason then that there is only one way to attain to that freedom which is the goal of all the noblest aspirations of mankind, and that is by giving up this little life, giving up this little universe, giving up this earth, giving up heaven, giving up the body, giving up the mind, giving up everything that is limited and conditioned.

If we give up our attachment to this little universe of the senses or of the mind, we shall be free immediately. The only way to come out of bondage is to go beyond the limitations of law, to go beyond causation.

But it is a most difficult thing to give up the clinging to this universe; few ever attain to that. There are two ways to do that mentioned in our books. One is called the "Neti, Neti" (not this, not this), the other is called "Iti" (this); the former is the negative, and the latter is the positive way.

The negative way is the most difficult. It is only possible to the men of the very highest, exceptional minds and gigantic wills who simply stand up and say, "No, I will not have this," and the mind and body obey their will, and they come out successful.

But such people are very rare. The vast majority of mankind choose the positive way, the way through the world, making use of all the bondages themselves to break those very bondages. This is also a kind of giving up; only it is done slowly and gradually, by knowing things, enjoying things and thus obtaining experience, and knowing the nature of things until the mind lets them all go at last and becomes unattached.

The former way of obtaining non-attachment is by reasoning, and the latter way is through work and experience. The first is the path of Jnâna-Yoga, and is characterized by the refusal to do any work; the second is that of Karma-Yoga, in which there is no cessation from work.

Every one must work in the universe. Only those who are perfectly satisfied with the Self, whose desires do not go beyond the Self, whose mind never strays out of the Self, to whom the Self is all in all, only those do not work. The rest must work.

A current rushing down of its own nature falls into a hollow and makes a whirlpool, and, after running a little in that whirlpool, it emerges again in the form of the free current to go on unchecked.

Each human life is like that current. It gets into the whirl, gets involved in this world of space, time, and causation, whirls round a little, crying out, "my father, my brother, my name, my fame", and so on, and at last emerges out of it and regains its original freedom.

The whole universe is doing that. Whether we know it or not, whether we are conscious or unconscious of it, we are all working to get out of the dream of the world. Man's experience in the world is to enable him to get out of its whirlpool.

What is Karma-Yoga? The knowledge of the secret of work. We see that the whole universe is working. For what? For salvation, for liberty; from the atom to the highest being, working for the one end, liberty for the mind, for the body, for the spirit.

All things are always trying to get freedom, flying away from bondage. The sun, the moon, the earth, the planets, all are trying to fly away from bondage. The centrifugal and the centripetal forces of nature are indeed typical of our universe. Instead of being knocked about in this universe, and after long delay and thrashing, getting to know things as they are, we learn from Karma-Yoga the secret of work, the method of work, the organising power of work.

A vast mass of energy may be spent in vain if we do not know how to utilise it. Karma-Yoga makes a science of work; you learn by it how best to utilise all the workings of this world. Work is inevitable, it must be so; but we should work to the highest purpose.

Karma-Yoga makes us admit that this world is a world of five minutes, that it is a something we have to pass through; and that freedom is not here, but is only to be found beyond. To find the way out of the bondages of the world we have to go through it slowly and surely.

There may be those exceptional persons about whom I just spoke, those who can stand aside and give up the world, as a snake casts off its skin and stands aside and looks at it. There are no doubt these exceptional beings; but the rest of mankind have to go slowly through the world of work. Karma-Yoga shows the process, the secret, and the method of doing it to the best advantage.

What does it say? "Work incessantly, but give up all attachment to work." Do not identify yourself with anything. Hold your mind free. All this that you see, the pains and the miseries, are but the necessary conditions of this world; poverty and wealth and happiness are but momentary; they do not belong to our real nature at all.

Our nature is far beyond misery and happiness, beyond every object of the senses, beyond the imagination; and yet we must go on working all the time. "Misery comes through attachment, not through work." As soon as we identify ourselves with the work we do, we feel miserable; but if we do not identify ourselves with it, we do not feel that misery.

If a beautiful picture belonging to another is burnt, a man does not generally become miserable; but when his own picture is burnt, how miserable he feels! Why? Both were beautiful pictures, perhaps copies of the same original; but in one case very much more misery is felt than in the other.

It is because in one case he identifies himself with the picture, and not in the other. This "I and mine" causes the whole misery. With the sense of possession comes selfishness, and selfishness brings on misery.

Every act of selfishness or thought of selfishness makes us attached to something, and immediately we are made slaves. Each wave in the Chitta that says "I and mine" immediately puts a chain round us and makes us slaves; and the more we say "I and mine", the more slavery grows, the more misery increases.

Therefore Karma-Yoga tells us to enjoy the beauty of all the pictures in the world, but not to identify ourselves with any of them. Never say "mine". Whenever we say a thing is "mine", misery will immediately come.

Do not even say "my child" in your mind. Possess the child, but do not say "mine". If you do, then will come the misery. Do not say "my house," do not say "my body".

The whole difficulty is there. The body is neither yours, nor mine, nor anybody's. These bodies are coming and going by the laws of nature, but we are free, standing as witness. This body is no more free than a picture or a wall.

Why should we be attached so much to a body? If somebody paints a picture, he does it and passes on. Do not project that tentacle of selfishness, "I must possess it". As soon as that is projected, misery will begin.

So Karma-Yoga says, first destroy the tendency to project this tentacle of selfishness, and when you have the power of checking it, hold it in and do not allow the mind to get into the ways of selfishness. Then you may go out into the world and work as much as you can.

Mix everywhere, go where you please; you will never be contaminated with evil. There is the lotus leaf in the water; the water cannot touch and adhere to it; so will you be in the world. This is called "Vairâgya", dispassion or non-attachment.

I believe I have told you that without non-attachment there cannot be any kind of Yoga. Non-attachment is the basis of all the Yogas. The man who gives up living in houses, wearing fine clothes, and eating good food, and goes into the desert, may be a most attached person. His only possession, his own body, may become everything to him; and as he lives he will be simply struggling for the sake of his body.

Non-attachment does not mean anything that we may do in relation to our external body, it is all in the mind. The binding link of "I and mine" is in the mind. If we have not this link with the body and with the things of the senses, we are non-attached, wherever and whatever we may be. A man may be on a throne and perfectly non-attached; another man may be in rags and still very much attached. First, we have to attain this state of non-attachment and then to work incessantly. Karma-Yoga gives us the method that will help us in giving up all attachment, though it is indeed very hard.

Here are the two ways of giving up all attachment. The one is for those who do not believe in God, or in any outside help. They are left to their own devices; they have simply to work with their own will, with the powers of their mind and discrimination, saying, "I must be non-attached".

For those who believe in God there is another way, which is much less difficult. They give up the fruits of work unto the Lord; they work and are never attached to the results. Whatever they see, feel, hear, or do, is for Him. For whatever good work we may do, let us not claim any praise or benefit. It is the Lord's; give up the fruits unto Him.

Let us stand aside and think that we are only servants obeying the Lord, our Master, and that every impulse for action comes from Him every moment. Whatever thou worshippest, whatever thou perceivest, whatever thou doest, give up all unto Him and be at rest.

Let us be at peace, perfect peace, with ourselves, and give up our whole body and mind and everything as an eternal sacrifice unto the Lord. Instead of the sacrifice of pouring oblations into the fire, perform this one great sacrifice day and night — the sacrifice of your little self.

"In search of wealth in this world, Thou art the only wealth I have found; I sacrifice myself unto Thee. In search of some one to be loved, Thou art the only one beloved I have found; I sacrifice myself unto Thee." Let us repeat this day and night, and say, "Nothing for me; no matter whether the thing is good, bad, or indifferent; I do not care for it; I sacrifice all unto Thee."

Day and night let us renounce our seeming self until it becomes a habit with us to do so, until it gets into the blood, the nerves, and the brain, and the whole body is every moment obedient to this idea of self-renunciation. Go then into the midst of the battlefield, with the roaring cannon and the din of war, and you will find yourself to be free and at peace.

Karma-Yoga teaches us that the ordinary idea of duty is on the lower plane; nevertheless, all of us have to do our duty. Yet we may see that this peculiar sense of duty is very often a great cause of misery.

Duty becomes a disease with us; it drags us ever forward. It catches hold of us and makes our whole life miserable. It is the bane of human life. This duty, this idea of duty is the midday summer sun which scorches the innermost soul of mankind.

Look at those poor slaves to duty! Duty leaves them no time to say prayers, no time to bathe. Duty is ever on them. They go out and work. Duty is on them! They come home and think of the work for the next day.

Duty is on them! It is living a slave's life, at last dropping down in the street and dying in harness, like a horse. This is duty as it is understood.

The only true duty is to be unattached and to work as free beings, to give up all work unto God. All our duties are His. Blessed are we that we are ordered out here. We serve our time; whether we do it ill or well, who knows? If we do it well, we do not get the fruits. If we do it ill, neither do we get the care. Be at rest, be free, and work.

This kind of freedom is a very hard thing to attain. How easy it is to interpret slavery as duty — the morbid attachment of flesh for flesh as duty! Men go out into the world and struggle and fight for money or for any other thing to which they get attached. Ask them why they do it. They say, "It is a duty". It is the absurd greed for gold and gain, and they try to cover it with a few flowers.

What is duty after all? It is really the impulsion of the flesh, of our attachment; and when an attachment has become established, we call it duty.

For instance, in countries where there is no marriage, there is no duty between husband and wife; when marriage comes, husband and wife live together on account of attachment; and that kind of living together becomes settled after generations; and when it becomes so settled, it becomes a duty. It is, so to say, a sort of chronic disease. When it is acute, we call it disease; when it is chronic, we call it nature. It is a disease.

So when attachment becomes chronic, we baptise it with the high sounding name of duty. We strew flowers upon it, trumpets sound for it, sacred texts are said over it, and then the whole world fights, and men earnestly rob each other for this duty's sake.

Duty is good to the extent that it checks brutality. To the lowest kinds of men, who cannot have any other ideal, it is of some good; but those who want to be Karma-Yogis must throw this idea of duty overboard. There is no duty for you and me. Whatever you have to give to the world, do give by all means, but not as a duty. Do not take any thought of that.

Be not compelled. Why should you be compelled? Everything that you do under compulsion goes to build up attachment. Why should you have any duty? Resign everything unto God. In this tremendous fiery furnace where the fire of duty scorches everybody, drink this cup of nectar and be happy. We are all simply working out His will, and have nothing to do with rewards and punishments.

If you want the reward, you must also have the punishment; the only way to get out of the punishment is to give up the reward. The only way of getting out of misery is by giving up the idea of happiness, because these two are linked to each other.

On one side there is happiness, on the other there is misery. On one side there is life, on the other there is death. The only way to get beyond death is to give up the love of life. Life and death are the same thing, looked at from different points.

So the idea of happiness without misery, or of life without death, is very good for school-boys and children; but the thinker sees that it is all a contradiction in terms and gives up both. Seek no praise, no reward, for anything you do.

No sooner do we perform a good action than we begin to desire credit for it. No sooner do we give money to some charity than we want to see our names blazoned in the papers. Misery must come as the result of such desires. The greatest men in the world have passed away unknown.

The Buddhas and the Christs that we know are but second-rate heroes in comparison with the greatest men of whom the world knows nothing. Hundreds of these unknown heroes have lived in every country working silently. Silently they live and silently they pass away; and in time their thoughts find expression in Buddhas or Christs, and it is these latter that become known to us.

The highest men do not seek to get any name or fame from their knowledge. They leave their ideas to the world; they put forth no claims for themselves and establish no schools or systems in their name. Their whole nature shrinks from such a thing. They are the pure Sâttvikas, who can never make any stir, but only melt down in love.

I have seen one such Yogi who lives in a cave in India. He is one of the most wonderful men I have ever seen. He has so completely lost the sense of his own individuality that we may say that the man in him is completely gone, leaving behind only the all comprehending sense of the divine.

If an animal bites one of his arms, he is ready to give it his other arm also, and say that it is the Lord's will. Everything that comes to him is from the Lord. He does not show himself to men, and yet he is a magazine of love and of true and sweet ideas.

Next in order come the men with more Rajas, or activity, combative natures, who take up the ideas of the perfect ones and preach them to the world. The highest kind of men silently collect true and noble ideas, and others — the Buddhas and Christs — go from place to place preaching them and working for them.

In the life of Gautama Buddha we notice him constantly saying that he is the twenty-fifth Buddha. The twenty-four before him are unknown to history, although the Buddha known to history must have built upon foundations laid by them.

The highest men are calm, silent, and unknown. They are the men who really know the power of thought; they are sure that, even if they go into a cave and close the door and simply think five true thoughts and then pass away, these five thoughts of theirs will live through eternity.

Indeed such thoughts will penetrate through the mountains, cross the oceans, and travel through the world. They will enter deep into human hearts and brains and raise up men and women who will give them practical expression in the workings of human life. These Sattvika men are too near the Lord to be active and to fight, to be working, struggling, preaching and doing good, as they say, here on earth to humanity.

The active workers, however good, have still a little remnant of ignorance left in them. When our nature has yet some impurities left in it, then alone can we work. It is in the nature of work to be impelled ordinarily by motive and by attachment.

In the presence of an ever active Providence who notes even the sparrow's fall, how can man attach any importance to his own work? Will it not be a blasphemy to do so when we know that He is taking care of the minutest things in the world? We have only to stand in awe and reverence before Him saying, "Thy will be done".

The highest men cannot work, for in them there is no attachment. Those whose whole soul is gone into the Self, those whose desires are confined in the Self, who have become ever associated with the Self, for them there is no work. Such are indeed the highest of mankind; but apart from them every one else has to work.

In so working we should never think that we can help on even the least thing in this universe. We cannot. We only help ourselves in this gymnasium of the world. This is the proper attitude of work.

If we work in this way, if we always remember that our present opportunity to work thus is a privilege which has been given to us, we shall never be attached to anything. Millions like you and me think that we are great people in the world; but we all die, and in five minutes the world forgets us.

But the life of God is infinite. "Who can live a moment, breathe a moment, if this all-powerful One does not will it?" He is the ever active Providence. All power is His and within His command. Through His command the winds blow, the sun shines, the earth lives, and death stalks upon the earth. He is the all in all; He is all and in all.

We can only worship Him. Give up all fruits of work; do good for its own sake; then alone will come perfect non-attachment. The bonds of the heart will thus break, and we shall reap perfect freedom. This freedom is indeed the goal of Karma-Yoga.

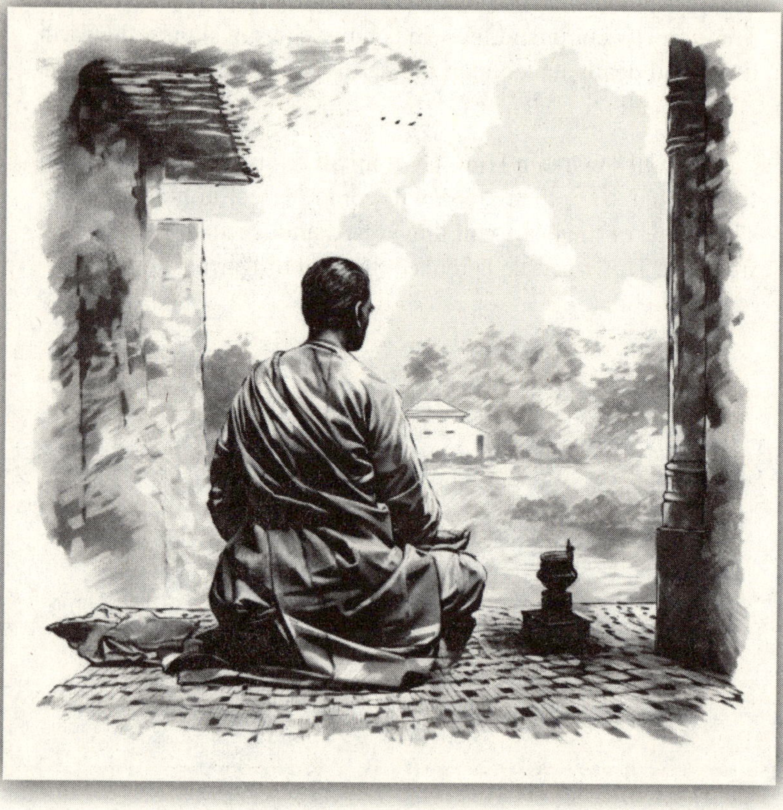

# The Karma-Yogi

Karma-Yoga is purifying the mind by means of work. Now if any work is done, good or bad, it must produce as a result a good or bad effect; no power can stay it, once the cause is present.

Therefore good action producing good Karma, and bad action, bad Karma, the soul will go on in eternal bondage without ever hoping for deliverance. Now Karma belongs only to the body or the mind, never to the Atman (Self); only it can cast a veil before the Atman.

The veil cast by bad Karma is ignorance. Good Karma has the power to strengthen the moral powers. And thus it creates non-attachment; it destroys the tendency towards bad Karma and thereby purifies the mind. But if the work is done with the intention of enjoyment, it then produces only that very enjoyment and does not purify the mind or Chitta.

Therefore all work should be done without any desire to enjoy the fruits thereof. All fear and all desire to enjoy here or hereafter must be banished for ever by the Karma-Yogi.

Moreover, this Karma without desire of return will destroy the selfishness, which is the root of all bondage. The watchword of the Karma-Yogi is "not I, but Thou", and no amount of self-sacrifice is too much for him. But he does this without any desire to go to heaven, or gain name or fame or any other benefit in this world.

Although the explanation and rationale of this unselfish work is only in Jnâna-Yoga, yet the natural divinity of man makes him love all sacrifice simply for the good of others, without any ulterior motive, whatever his creed or opinion. Again, with many the bondage of wealth is very great; and Karma-Yoga is absolutely necessary for them as breaking the crystallisation that has gathered round their love of money.

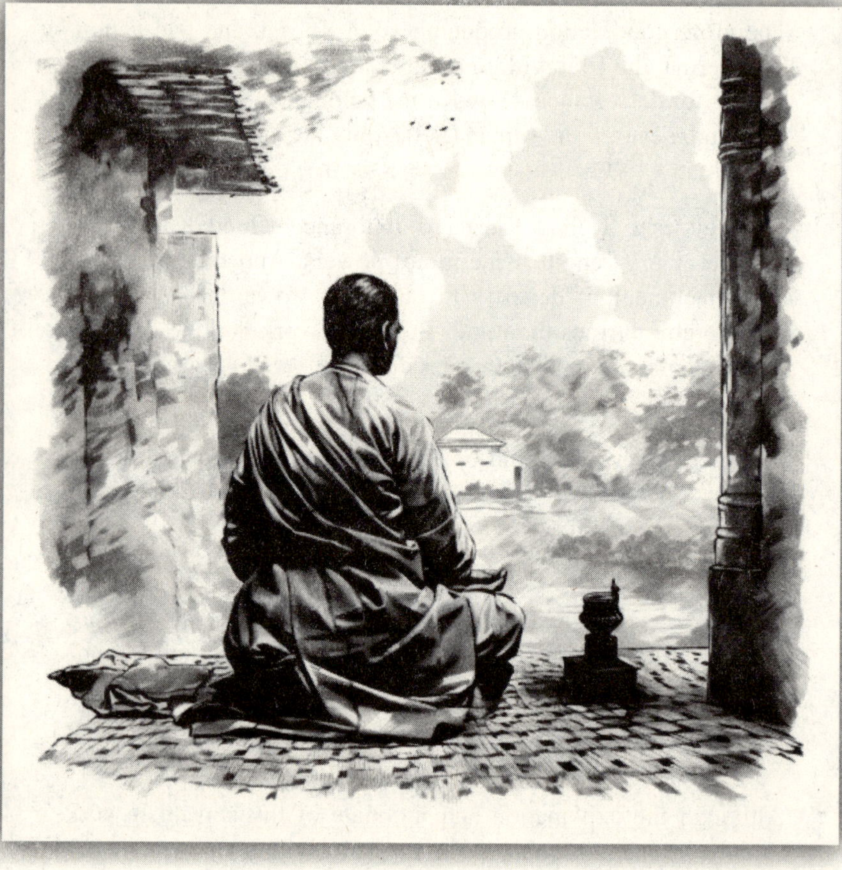

# The Ideal Of Karma-Yoga

The grandest idea in the religion of the Vedanta is that we may reach the same goal by different paths; and these paths I have generalised into four, viz those of work, love, psychology, and knowledge. But you must, at the same time, remember that these divisions are not very marked and quite exclusive of each other. Each blends into the other.

But according to the type which prevails, we name the divisions. It is not that you can find men who have no other faculty than that of work, nor that you can find men who are no more than devoted worshippers only, nor that there are men who have no more than mere knowledge.

These divisions are made in accordance with the type or the tendency that may be seen to prevail in a man. We have found that, in the end, all these four paths converge and become one. All religions and all methods of work and worship lead us to one and the same goal.

I have already tried to point out that goal. It is freedom as I understand it. Everything that we perceive around us is struggling towards freedom, from the atom to the man, from the insentient, lifeless particle of matter to the highest existence on earth, the human soul.

The whole universe is in fact the result of this struggle for freedom. In all combinations every particle is trying to go on its own way, to fly from the other particles; but the others are holding it in check. Our earth is trying to fly away from the sun, and the moon from the earth. Everything has a tendency to infinite dispersion. All that we see in the universe has for its basis this one struggle towards freedom; it is under the impulse of this tendency that the saint prays and the robber robs.

When the line of action taken is not a proper one, we call it evil; and when the manifestation of it is proper and high, we call it good. But the impulse is the same, the struggle towards freedom. The saint is oppressed with the knowledge of his condition of bondage, and he wants to get rid of it; so he worships God. The thief is oppressed with the idea that he does not possess certain things, and he tries to get rid of that want, to obtain freedom from it; so he steals.

Freedom is the one goal of all nature, sentient or insentient; and consciously or unconsciously, everything is struggling towards that goal. The freedom which the saint seeks is very different from that which the robber seeks; the freedom loved by the saint leads him to the enjoyment of infinite, unspeakable bliss, while that on which the robber has set his heart only forges other bonds for his soul.

There is to be found in every religion the manifestation of this struggle towards freedom. It is the groundwork of all morality, of unselfishness, which means getting rid of the idea that men are the same as their little body.

When we see a man doing good work, helping others, it means that he cannot be confined within the limited circle of "me and mine". There is no limit to this getting out of selfishness. All the great systems of ethics preach absolute unselfishness as the goal.

Supposing this absolute unselfishness can be reached by a man, what becomes of him? He is no more the little Mr. So-and-so; he has acquired infinite expansion. The little personality which he had before is now lost to him for ever; he has become infinite, and the attainment of this infinite expansion is indeed the goal of all religions and of all moral and philosophical teachings.

The personalist, when he hears this idea philosophically put, gets frightened. At the same time, if he preaches morality, he after all teaches the very same idea himself. He puts no limit to the unselfishness of man.

Suppose a man becomes perfectly unselfish under the personalistic system, how are we to distinguish him from the perfected ones in other system? He has become one with the universe and to become that is the goal of all; only the poor personalist has not the courage to follow out his own reasoning to its right conclusion. Karma-Yoga is the attaining through unselfish work of that freedom which is the goal of all human nature.

Every selfish action, therefore, retards our reaching the goal, and every unselfish action takes us towards the goal; that is why the only definition that can be given of morality is this: That which is selfish is immoral, and that which is unselfish is moral.

But, if you come to details, the matter will not be seen to be quite so simple. For instance, environment often makes the details different as I have already mentioned. The same action under one set of circumstances may be unselfish, and under another set quite selfish.

So we can give only a general definition, and leave the details to be worked out by taking into consideration the differences in time, place, and circumstances. In one country one kind of conduct is considered moral, and in another the very same is immoral, because the circumstances differ.

The goal of all nature is freedom, and freedom is to be attained only by perfect unselfishness; every thought, word, or deed that is unselfish takes us towards the goal, and, as such, is called moral. That definition, you will find, holds good in every religion and every system of ethics. In some systems of thought morality is derived from a Superior Being — God.

If you ask why a man ought to do this and not that, their answer is: "Because such is the command of God." But whatever be the source from which it is derived, their code of ethics also has the same central idea — not to think of self but to give up self.

And yet some persons, in spite of this high ethical idea, are frightened at the thought of having to give up their little personalities. We may ask the man who clings to the idea of little personalities to consider the case of a person who has become perfectly unselfish, who has no thought for himself, who does no deed for himself, who speaks no word for himself, and then say where his "himself" is.

That "himself" is known to him only so long as he thinks, acts, or speaks for himself. If he is only conscious of others, of the universe, and of the all, where is his "himself"? It is gone for ever.

Karma-Yoga, therefore, is a system of ethics and religion intended to attain freedom through unselfishness, and by good works. The Karma-Yogi need not believe in any doctrine whatever. He may not believe even in God, may not ask what his soul is, nor think of any metaphysical speculation. He has got his own special aim of realising selflessness; and he has to work it out himself.

Every moment of his life must be realisation, because he has to solve by mere work, without the help of doctrine or theory, the very same problem to which the Jnâni applies his reason and inspiration and the Bhakta his love.

Now comes the next question: What is this work? What is this doing good to the world? Can we do good to the world? In an absolute sense, no; in a relative sense, yes. No permanent or everlasting good can be done to the world; if it could be done, the world would not be this world. We may satisfy the hunger of a man for five minutes, but he will be hungry again. Every pleasure with which we supply a man may be seen to be momentary. No one can permanently cure this ever-recurring fever of pleasure and pain.

Can any permanent happiness be given to the world? In the ocean we cannot raise a wave without causing a hollow somewhere else. The sum total of the good things in the world has been the same throughout in its relation to man's need and greed. It cannot be increased or decreased.

Take the history of the human race as we know it today. Do we not find the same miseries and the same happiness, the same pleasures and pains, the same differences in position? Are not some rich, some poor, some high, some low, some healthy, some unhealthy?

All this was just the same with the Egyptians, the Greeks, and the Romans in ancient times as it is with the Americans today. So far as history is known, it has always been the same; yet at the same time we find that, running along with all these incurable differences of pleasure and pain, there has ever been the struggle to alleviate them.

Every period of history has given birth to thousands of men and women who have worked hard to smooth the passage of life for others. And how far have they succeeded? We can only play at driving the ball from one place to another. We take away pain from the physical plane, and it goes to the mental one.

It is like that picture in Dante's hell where the misers were given a mass of gold to roll up a hill. Every time they rolled it up a little, it again rolled down. All our talks about the millennium are very nice as school-boys' stories, but they are no better than that. All nations that dream of the millennium also think that, of all peoples in the world, they will have the best of it then for themselves. This is the wonderfully unselfish idea of the millennium!

We cannot add happiness to this world; similarly, we cannot add pain to it either. The sum total of the energies of pleasure and pain displayed here on earth will be the same throughout. We just push it from this side to the other side, and from that side to this, but it will remain the same, because to remain so is its very nature. This ebb and flow, this rising and falling, is in the world's very nature; it would be as logical to hold otherwise as to say that we may have life without death.

This is complete nonsense, because the very idea of life implies death and the very idea of pleasure implies pain. The lamp is constantly burning out, and that is its life. If you want to have life, you have to die every moment for it.

Life and death are only different expressions of the same thing looked at from different standpoints; they are the falling and the rising of the same wave, and the two form one whole. One looks at the "fall" side and becomes a pessimist another looks at the "rise" side and becomes an optimist.

When a boy is going to school and his father and mother are taking care of him, everything seems blessed to him; his wants are simple, he is a great optimist. But the old man, with his varied experience, becomes calmer and is sure to have his warmth considerably cooled down. So, old nations, with signs of decay all around them, are apt to be less hopeful than new nations.

There is a proverb in India: "A thousand years a city, and a thousand years a forest." This change of city into forest and vice versa is going on everywhere, and it makes people optimists or pessimists according to the side they see of it.

The next idea we take up is the idea of equality. These millennium ideas have been great motive powers to work. Many religions preach this as an element in them — that God is coming to rule the universe, and that then there will be no difference at all in conditions.

The people who preach this doctrine are mere fanatics, and fanatics are indeed the sincerest of mankind. Christianity was preached just on the basis of the fascination of this fanaticism, and that is what made it so attractive to the Greek and the Roman slaves. They believed that under the millennial religion there would be no more slavery, that there would be plenty to eat and drink; and, therefore, they flocked round the Christian standard. Those who preached the idea first were of course ignorant fanatics, but very sincere.

In modern times this millennial aspiration takes the form of equality — of liberty, equality, and fraternity. This is also fanaticism. True equality has never been and never can be on earth. How can we all be equal here? This impossible kind of equality implies total death.

What makes this world what it is? Lost balance. In the primal state, which is called chaos, there is perfect balance. How do all the formative forces of the universe come then? By struggling, competition, conflict.

Suppose that all the particles of matter were held in equilibrium, would there be then any process of creation? We know from science that it is impossible. Disturb a sheet of water, and there you find every particle of the water trying to become calm again, one rushing against the other; and in the same way all the phenomena which we call the universe — all things therein — are struggling to get back to the state of perfect balance. Again a disturbance comes, and again we have combination and creation.

Inequality is the very basis of creation. At the same time the forces struggling to obtain equality are as much a necessity of creation as those which destroy it.

Absolute equality, that which means a perfect balance of all the struggling forces in all the planes, can never be in this world. Before you attain that state, the world will have become quite unfit for any kind of life, and no one will be there. We find, therefore, that all these ideas of the millennium and of absolute equality are not only impossible but also that, if we try to carry them out, they will lead us surely enough to the day of destruction.

What makes the difference between man and man? It is largely the difference in the brain. Nowadays no one but a lunatic will say that we are all born with the same brain power. We come into the world with unequal endowments; we come as greater men or as lesser men, and there is no getting away from that pre-natally determined condition.

The American Indians were in this country for thousands of years, and a few handfuls of your ancestors came to their land. What difference they have caused in the appearance of the country! Why did not the Indians make improvements and build cities, if all were equal? With your ancestors a different sort of brain power came into the land, different bundles of past impressions came, and they worked out and manifested themselves.

Absolute non-differentiation is death. So long as this world lasts, differentiation there will and must be, and the millennium of perfect equality will come only when a cycle of creation comes to its end. Before that, equality cannot be.

Yet this idea of realising the millennium is a great motive power. Just as inequality is necessary for creation itself, so the struggle to limit it is also necessary. If there were no struggle to become free and get back to God, there would be no creation either. It is the difference between these two forces that determines the nature of the motives of men. There will always be these motives to work, some tending towards bondage and others towards freedom.

This world's wheel within wheel is a terrible mechanism; if we put our hands in it, as soon as we are caught we are gone. We all think that when we have done a certain duty, we shall be at rest; but before we have done a part of that duty, another is already in waiting. We are all being dragged along by this mighty, complex world-machine.

There are only two ways out of it; one is to give up all concerns with the machine, to let it go and stand aside, to give up our desires. That is very easy to say, but is almost impossible to do. I do not know whether in twenty millions of men one can do that.

The other way is to plunge into the world and learn the secret of work, and that is the way of Karma-Yoga. Do not fly away from the wheels of the world-machine, but stand inside it and learn the secret of work. Through proper work done inside, it is also possible to come out. Through this machinery itself is the way out.

We have now seen what work is. It is a part of natures foundation, and goes on always. Those that believe in God understand this better, because they know that God is not such an incapable being as will need our help.

Although this universe will go on always, our goal is freedom, our goal is unselfishness; and according to Karma-Yoga, that goal is to be reached through work. All ideas of making the world perfectly happy may be good as motive powers for fanatics; but we must know that fanaticism brings forth as much evil as good.

The Karma-Yogi asks why you require any motive to work other than the inborn love of freedom. Be beyond the common worldly motives. "To work you have the right, but not to the fruits thereof." Man can train himself to know and to practice that, says the Karma-Yogi.

When the idea of doing good becomes a part of his very being, then he will not seek for any motive outside. Let us do good because it is good to do good; he who does good work even in order to get to heaven binds himself down, says the Karma-Yogi. Any work that is done with any the least selfish motive, instead of making us free, forges one more chain for our feet.

So the only way is to give up all the fruits of work, to be unattached to them. Know that this world is not we, nor are we this world; that we are really not the body; that we really do not work. We are the Self, eternally at rest and at peace.

Why should we be bound by anything? It is very good to say that we should be perfectly non-attached, but what is the way to do it? Every good work we do without any ulterior motive, instead of forging a new chain, will break one of the links in the existing chains. Every good thought that we send to the world without thinking of any return, will be stored up there and break one link in the chain, and make us purer and purer, until we become the purest of mortals.

Yet all this may seem to be rather quixotic and too philosophical, more theoretical than practical. I have read many arguments against the Bhagavad-Gita, and many have said that without motives you cannot work. They have never seen unselfish work except under the influence of fanaticism, and, therefore, they speak in that way.

It is evident that in society there are many persons who seem to be born for some sort of activity or other, whose minds cannot be concentrated on the plane of thought alone, and who have but one idea, concretised in work, visible and tangible. There must be a science for this kind of life too.

Each one of us is engaged in some work, but the majority of us fritter away the greater portion of our energies, because we do not know the secret of work. Karma-Yoga explains this secret and teaches where and how to work, how to employ to the greatest advantage the largest part of our energies in the work that is before us.

But with this secret we must take into consideration the great objection against work, namely that it causes pain. All misery and pain come from attachment.

I want to do work, I want to do good to a human being; and it is ninety to one that that human being whom I have helped will prove ungrateful and go against me; and the result to me is pain. Such things deter mankind from working; and it spoils a good portion of the work and energy of mankind, this fear of pain and misery.

Karma-Yoga teaches us how to work for work's sake, unattached, without caring who is helped, and what for. The Karma-Yogi works because it is his nature, because he feels that it is good for him to do so, and he has no object beyond that.

His position in this world is that of a giver, and he never cares to receive anything. He knows that he is giving, and does not ask for anything in return and, therefore, he eludes the grasp of misery. The grasp of pain, whenever it comes, is the result of the reaction of "attachment".

Let me tell you in conclusion a few words about one man who actually carried this teaching of Karma-Yoga into practice. That man is Buddha. He is the one man who ever carried this into perfect practice.

All the prophets of the world, except Buddha, had external motives to move them to unselfish action. The prophets of the world, with this single exception, may be divided into two sets, one set holding that they are incarnations of God come down on earth, and the other holding that they are only messengers from God; and both draw their impetus for work from outside, expect reward from outside, however highly spiritual may be the language they use.

But Buddha is the only prophet who said, "I do not care to know your various theories about God. What is the use of discussing all the subtle doctrines about the soul? Do good and be good. And this will take you to freedom and to whatever truth there is."

He was, in the conduct of his life, absolutely without personal motives; and what man worked more than he? Show me in history one character who has soared so high above all. The whole human race has produced but one such character, such high philosophy, such wide sympathy. This great philosopher, preaching the highest philosophy, yet had the deepest sympathy for the lowest of animals, and never put forth any claims for himself.

He is the ideal Karma-Yogi, acting entirely without motive, and the history of humanity shows him to have been the greatest man ever born; beyond compare the greatest combination of heart and brain that ever existed, the greatest soul-power that has even been manifested.

He is the first great reformer the world has seen. He was the first who dared to say, "Believe not because some old manuscripts are produced, believe not because it is your national belief, because you have been made to believe it from your childhood; but reason it all out, and after you have analysed it, then, if you find that it will do good to one and all, believe it, live up to it, and help others to live up to it."

He works best who works without any motive, neither for money, nor for fame, nor for anything else; and when a man can do that, he will be a Buddha, and out of him will come the power to work in such a manner as will transform the world. This man represents the very highest ideal of Karma-Yoga.

# Raja

# The Power of the Mind

All over the world there has been the belief in the supernatural throughout the ages. All of us have heard of extraordinary happenings, and many of us have had some personal experience of them. I would rather introduce the subject by telling you certain facts which have come within my own experience.

I once heard of a man who, if any one went to him with questions in his mind, would answer them immediately; and I was also informed that he foretold events. I was curious and went to see him with a few friends. We each had something in our minds to ask, and, to avoid mistakes, we wrote down our questions and put them in our pockets.

As soon as the man saw one of us, he repeated our questions and gave the answers to them. Then he wrote something on paper, which he folded up, asked me to sign on the back, and said, "Don't look at it; put it in your pocket and keep it there till I ask for it again." And so on to each one of us.

He next told us about some events that would happen to us in the future. Then he said, "Now, think of a word or a sentence, from any language you like."

I thought of a long sentence from Sanskrit, a language of which he was entirely ignorant. "Now, take out the paper from your pocket," he said.

The Sanskrit sentence was written there! He had written it an hour before with the remark, "In confirmation of what I have written, this man will think of this sentence."

It was correct. Another of us who had been given a similar paper which he had signed and placed in his pocket, was also asked to think of a sentence. He thought of a sentence in Arabic, which it was still less possible for the man to know; it was some passage from the Koran. And my friend found this written down on the paper.

Another of us was a physician. He thought of a sentence from a German medical book. It was written on his paper.

Several days later I went to this man again, thinking possibly I had been deluded somehow before. I took other friends, and on this occasion also he came out wonderfully triumphant.

Another time I was in the city of Hyderabad in India, and I was told of a Brâhmin there who could produce numbers of things from where, nobody knew. This man was in business there; he was a respectable gentleman. And I asked him to show me his tricks.

It so happened that this man had a fever, and in India there is a general belief that if a holy man puts his hand on a sick man he would be well. This Brahmin came to me and said, "Sir, put your hand on my head, so that my fever may be cured."

I said, "Very good; but you show me your tricks."

He promised. I put my hand on his head as desired, and later he came to fulfil his promise. He had only a strip of cloth about his loins, we took off everything else from him. I had a blanket which I gave him to wrap round himself, because it was cold, and made him sit in a corner. Twenty-five pairs of eyes were looking at him.

And he said, "Now, look, write down anything you want."

We all wrote down names of fruits that never grew in that country, bunches of grapes, oranges, and so on. And we gave him those bits of paper.

And there came from under his blanket, bushels of grapes, oranges, and so forth, so much that if all that fruit was weighed, it would have been twice as heavy as the man. He asked us to eat the fruit. Some of us objected, thinking it was hypnotism; but the man began eating himself — so we all ate. It was all right.

He ended by producing a mass of roses. Each flower was perfect, with dew-drops on the petals, not one crushed, not one injured.

And masses of them! When I asked the man for an explanation, he said, "It is all sleight of hand."

Whatever it was, it seemed to be impossible that it could be sleight of hand merely. From whence could he have got such large quantities of things?

Well, I saw many things like that. Going about India you find hundreds of similar things in different places. These are in every country. Even in this country you will find some such wonderful things.

Of course, there is a great deal of fraud, no doubt; but then, whenever you see fraud, you have also to say that fraud is an imitation. There must be some truth somewhere, that is being imitated; you cannot imitate nothing. Imitation must be of something substantially true.

In very remote times in India, thousands of years ago, these facts used to happen even more than they do today. It seems to me that when a country becomes very thickly populated, psychical power deteriorates.

Given a vast country thinly inhabited, there will, perhaps, be more of psychical power there. These facts, the Hindus, being analytically minded. took up and investigated.

And they came to certain remarkable conclusions; that is, they made a science of it. They found out that all these, though extraordinary, are also natural; there is nothing supernatural. They are under laws just the same as any other physical phenomenon. It is not a freak of nature that a man is born with such powers. They can be systematically studied, practiced, and acquired.

This science they call the science of Râja-Yoga. There are thousands of people who cultivate the study of this science, and for the whole nation it has become a part of daily worship.

The conclusion they have reached is that all these extraordinary powers are in the mind of man. This mind is a part of the universal mind. Each mind is connected with every other mind. And each mind, wherever it is located, is in actual communication with the whole world.

Have you ever noticed the phenomenon that is called thought-transference? A man here is thinking something, and that thought is manifested in somebody else, in some other place. With preparations — not by chance — a man wants to send a thought to another mind at a distance, and this other mind knows that a thought is coming, and he receives it exactly as it is sent out.

Distance makes no difference. The thought goes and reaches the other man, and he understands it. If your mind were an isolated something here, and my mind were an isolated something there, and there were no connection between the two, how would it be possible for my thought to reach you?

In the ordinary cases, it is not my thought that is reaching you direct; but my thought has got to be dissolved into ethereal vibrations and those ethereal vibrations go into your brain, and they have to be resolved again into your own thoughts. Here is a dissolution of thought, and there is a resolution of thought. It is a roundabout process. But in telepathy, there is no such thing; it is direct.

This shows that there is a continuity of mind, as the Yogis call it. The mind is universal. Your mind, my mind, all these little minds, are fragments of that universal mind, little waves in the ocean; and on account of this continuity, we can convey our thoughts directly to one another.

You see what is happening all around us. The world is one of influence. Part of our energy is used up in the preservation of our own bodies. Beyond that, every particle of our energy is day and night being used in influencing others.

Our bodies, our virtues, our intellect, and our spirituality, all these are continuously influencing others; and so, conversely, we are being influenced by them. This is going on all around us.

Now, to take a concrete example. A man comes; you know he is very learned, his language is beautiful, and he speaks to you by the hour; but he does not make any impression.

Another man comes, and he speaks a few words, not well arranged, ungrammatical perhaps; all the same, he makes an immense impression. Many of you have seen that.

So it is evident that words alone cannot always produce an impression. Words, even thoughts contribute only one-third of the influence in making an impression, the man, two-thirds. What you call the personal magnetism of the man — that is what goes out and impresses you.

In our families there are the heads; some of them are successful, others are not. Why? We complain of others in our failures. The moment I am unsuccessful, I say, so-and-so is the cause of the failure.

In failure, one does not like to confess one's own faults and weaknesses. Each person tries to hold himself faultless and lay the blame upon somebody or something else, or even on bad luck.

When heads of families fail, they should ask themselves, why it is that some persons manage a family so well and others do not. Then you will find that the difference is owing to the man — his presence, his personality.

Coming to great leaders of mankind, we always find that it was the personality of the man that counted. Now, take all the great authors of the past, the great thinkers.

Really speaking, how many thoughts have they thought? Take all the writings that have been left to us by the past leaders of mankind; take each one of their books and appraise them. The real thoughts, new and genuine, that have been thought in this world up to this time, amount to only a handful.

Read in their books the thoughts they have left to us. The authors do not appear to be giants to us, and yet we know that they were great giants in their days. What made them so? Not simply the thoughts they thought, neither the books they wrote, nor the speeches they made, it was something else that is now gone, that is their personality.

The personality of the man is two-thirds, and his intellect, his words, are but one-third. It is the real man, the personality of the man, that runs through us. Our actions are but effects. Actions must come when the man is there; the effect is bound to follow the cause.

The ideal of all education, all training, should be this man-making. But, instead of that, we are always trying to polish up the outside. What use in polishing up the outside when there is no inside? The end and aim of all training is to make the man grow.

The man who influences, who throws his magic, as it were, upon his fellow-beings, is a dynamo of power, and when that man is ready, he can do anything and everything he likes; that personality put upon anything will make it work.

Now, we see that though this is a fact, no physical laws that we know of will explain this. How can we explain it by chemical and physical knowledge? How much of oxygen, hydrogen, carbon, how many molecules in different positions, and how many cells, etc., etc. can explain this mysterious personality?

And we still see, it is a fact, and not only that, it is the real man; and it is that man that lives and moves and works, it is that man that influences, moves his fellow-beings, and passes out, and his intellect and books and works are but traces left behind.

Think of this. Compare the great teachers of religion with the great philosophers. The philosophers scarcely influenced anybody's inner man, and yet they wrote most marvellous books. The religious teachers, on the other hand, moved countries in their lifetime.

The difference was made by personality. In the philosopher it is a faint personality that influences; in the great prophets it is tremendous. In the former we touch the intellect, in the latter we touch life. In the one case, it is simply a chemical process, putting certain chemical ingredients together which may gradually combine and under proper circumstances bring out a flash of light or may fail. In the other, it is like a torch that goes round quickly, lighting others.

The science of Yoga claims that it has discovered the laws which develop this personality, and by proper attention to those laws and methods, each one can grow and strengthen his personality. This is one of the great practical things, and this is the secret of all education.

This has a universal application. In the life of the householder, in the life of the poor, the rich, the man of business, the spiritual man, in every one's life, it is a great thing, the strengthening of this personality. There are laws, very fine, which are behind the physical laws, as we know.

That is to say, there are no such realities as a physical world, a mental world, a spiritual world. Whatever is, is one.

Let us say, it is a sort of tapering existence; the thickest part is here, it tapers and becomes finer and finer. The finest is what we call spirit; the grossest, the body. And just as it is here in microcosm, it is exactly the same in the macrocosm. The universe of ours is exactly like that; it is the gross external thickness, and it tapers into something finer and finer until it becomes God.

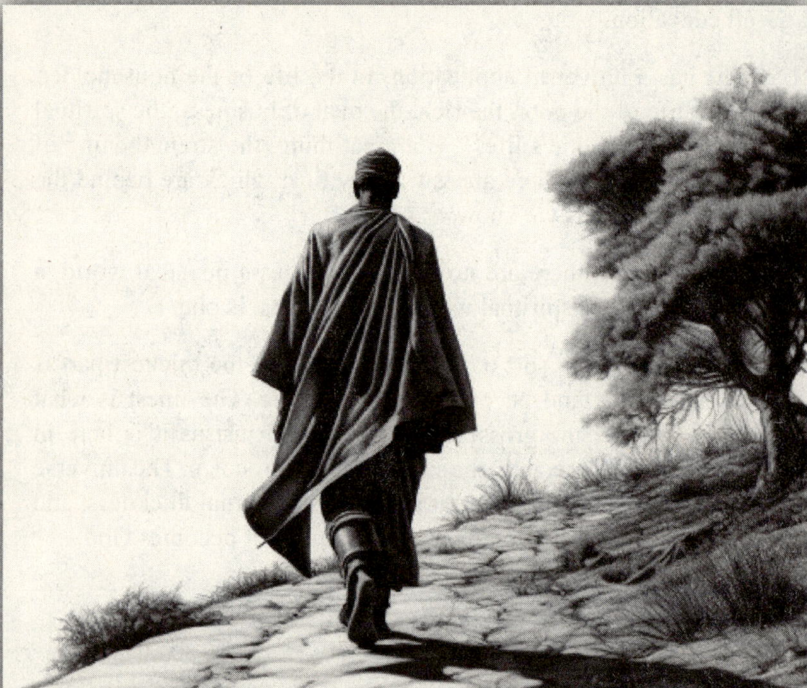

# The First Steps

Râja-Yoga is divided into eight steps.

The first is Yama — non-killing, truthfulness, non-stealing, continence, and non-receiving of any gifts. Next is Niyama — cleanliness, contentment, austerity, study, and self-surrender to God.

Then comes Âsana, or posture; Prânâyâma, or control of Prâna; Pratyâhâra, or restraint of the senses from their objects; Dhâranâ, or fixing the mind on a spot; Dhyâna, or meditation; and Samâdhi, or superconsciousness.

The Yama and Niyama, as we see, are moral trainings; without these as the basis no practice of Yoga will succeed. As these two become established, the Yogi will begin to realise the fruits of his practice; without these it will never bear fruit.

A Yogi must not think of injuring anyone, by thought, word, or deed. Mercy shall not be for men alone, but shall go beyond, and embrace the whole world.

The next step is Asana, posture. A series of exercises, physical and mental, is to be gone through every day, until certain higher states are reached. Therefore it is quite necessary that we should find a posture in which we can remain long.

That posture which is the easiest for one should be the one chosen. For thinking, a certain posture may be very easy for one man, while to another it may be very difficult. We will find later on that during the study of these psychological matters a good deal of activity goes on in the body.

Nerve currents will have to be displaced and given a new channel. New sorts of vibrations will begin, the whole constitution will be remodelled as it were.

But the main part of the activity will lie along the spinal column, so that the one thing necessary for the posture is to hold the spinal column free, sitting erect, holding the three parts — the chest, neck, and head — in a straight line. Let the whole weight of the body be supported by the ribs, and then you have an easy natural posture with the spine straight.

You will easily see that you cannot think very high thoughts with the chest in. This portion of the Yoga is a little similar to the Hatha-Yoga which deals entirely with the physical body, its aim being to make the physical body very strong. We have nothing to do with it here, because its practices are very difficult, and cannot be learned in a day, and, after all, do not lead to much spiritual growth.

Many of these practices you will find in Delsarte and other teachers, such as placing the body in different postures, but the object in these is physical, not psychological. There is not one muscle in the body over which a man cannot establish a perfect control. The heart can be made to stop or go on at his bidding, and each part of the organism can be similarly controlled.

The result of this branch of Yoga is to make men live long; health is the chief idea, the one goal of the Hatha-Yogi. He is determined not to fall sick, and he never does. He lives long; a hundred years is nothing to him; he is quite young and fresh when he is 150, without one hair turned grey.

But that is all. A banyan tree lives sometimes 5000 years, but it is a banyan tree and nothing more. So, if a man lives long, he is only a healthy animal.

One or two ordinary lessons of the Hatha-Yogis are very useful. For instance, some of you will find it a good thing for headaches to drink cold water through the nose as soon as you get up in the morning; the whole day your brain will be nice and cool, and you will never catch cold. It is very easy to do; put your nose into the water, draw it up through the nostrils and make a pump action in the throat.

After one has learned to have a firm erect seat, one has to perform, according to certain schools, a practice called the purifying of the nerves.

This part has been rejected by some as not belonging to Raja-Yoga, but as so great an authority as the commentator Shankarâchârya advises it, I think fit that it should be mentioned, and I will quote his own directions from his commentary on the Shvetâshvatara Upanishad:

"The mind whose dross has been cleared away by Pranayama, becomes fixed in Brahman; therefore Pranayama is declared.

"First the nerves are to be purified, then comes the power to practice Pranayama. Stopping the right nostril with the thumb, through the left nostril fill in air, according to capacity; then, without any interval, throw the air out through the right nostril, closing the left one.

"Again inhaling through the right nostril eject through the left, according to capacity; practicing this three or five times at four hours of the day, before dawn, during midday, in the evening, and at midnight, in fifteen days or a month purity of the nerves is attained; then begins Pranayama."

Practice is absolutely necessary. You may sit down and listen to me by the hour every day, but if you do not practice, you will not get one step further. It all depends on practice.

We never understand these things until we experience them. We will have to see and feel them for ourselves. Simply listening to explanations and theories will not do.

There are several obstructions to practice. The first obstruction is an unhealthy body: if the body is not in a fit state, the practice will be obstructed. Therefore we have to keep the body in good health; we have to take care of what we eat and drink, and what we do.

Always use a mental effort, what is usually called "Christian Science," to keep the body strong. That is all — nothing further of the body.

We must not forget that health is only a means to an end. If health were the end, we would be like animals; animals rarely become unhealthy.

The second obstruction is doubt; we always feel doubtful about things we do not see. Man cannot live upon words, however he may try. So, doubt comes to us as to whether there is any truth in these things or not; even the best of us will doubt sometimes: With practice, within a few days, a little glimpse will come, enough to give one encouragement and hope.

As a certain commentator on Yoga philosophy says, "When one proof is obtained, however little that may be, it will give us faith in the whole teaching of Yoga."

For instance, after the first few months of practice, you will begin to find you can read another's thoughts; they will come to you in picture form. Perhaps you will hear something happening at a long distance, when you concentrate your mind with a wish to hear. These glimpses will come, by little bits at first, but enough to give you faith, and strength, and hope.

For instance, if you concentrate your thoughts on the tip of your nose, in a few days you will begin to smell most beautiful fragrance, which will be enough to show you that there are certain mental perceptions that can be made obvious without the contact of physical objects.

But we must always remember that these are only the means; the aim, the end, the goal, of all this training is liberation of the soul. Absolute control of nature, and nothing short of it, must be the goal. We must be the masters, and not the slaves of nature; neither body nor mind must be our master, nor must we forget that the body is mine, and not I the body's.

A god and a demon went to learn about the Self from a great sage. They studied with him for a long time. At last the sage told them, "You yourselves are the Being you are seeking."

Both of them thought that their bodies were the Self. They went back to their people quite satisfied and said, "We have learned everything that was to be learned; eat, drink, and be merry; we are the Self; there is nothing beyond us."

The nature of the demon was ignorant, clouded; so he never inquired any further, but was perfectly contented with the idea that he was God, that by the Self was meant the body.

The god had a purer nature. He at first committed the mistake of thinking: I, this body, am Brahman: so keep it strong and in health, and well dressed, and give it all sorts of enjoyments.

But, in a few days, he found out that that could not be the meaning of the sage, their master; there must be something higher. So he came back and said, "Sir, did you teach me that this body was the Self? If so, I see all bodies die; the Self cannot die."

The sage said, "Find it out; thou art That."

Then the god thought that the vital forces which work the body were what the sage meant. But. after a time, he found that if he ate, these vital forces remained strong, but, if he starved, they became weak.

The god then went back to the sage and said, "Sir, do you mean that the vital forces are the Self ?"

The sage said, "Find out for yourself; thou art That."

The god returned home once more, thinking that it was the mind, perhaps, that was the Self. But in a short while he saw that thoughts were so various, now good, again bad; the mind was too changeable to be the Self. He went back to the sage and said, "Sir, I do not think that the mind is the Self; did you mean that?"

"No," replied the sage, "thou art That; find out for yourself."

The god went home, and at last found that he was the Self, beyond all thought, one without birth or death, whom the sword cannot pierce or the fire burn, whom the air cannot dry or the water melt, the beginningless and endless, the immovable, the intangible, the omniscient, the omnipotent Being; that It was neither the body nor the mind, but beyond them all.

So he was satisfied; but the poor demon did not get the truth, owing to his fondness for the body.

This world has a good many of these demoniac natures, but there are some gods too. If one proposes to teach any science to increase the power of sense-enjoyment, one finds multitudes ready for it. If one undertakes to show the supreme goal, one finds few to listen to him.

Very few have the power to grasp the higher, fewer still the patience to attain to it. But there are a few also who know that even if the body can be made to live for a thousand years, the result in the end will be the same. When the forces that hold it together go away, the body must fall. No man was ever born who could stop his body one moment from changing. Body is the name of a series of changes.

"As in a river the masses of water are changing before you every moment, and new masses are coming, yet taking similar form, so is it with this body."

Yet the body must be kept strong and healthy. It is the best instrument we have.

This human body is the greatest body in the universe, and a human being the greatest being. Man is higher than all animals, than all angels; none is greater than man. Even the Devas (gods) will have to come down again and attain to salvation through a human body.

Man alone attains to perfection, not even the Devas. According to the Jews and Mohammedans, God created man after creating the angels and everything else, and after creating man He asked the angels to come and salute him, and all did so except Iblis; so God cursed him and he became Satan.

Behind this allegory is the great truth that this human birth is the greatest birth we can have. The lower creation, the animal, is dull, and manufactured mostly out of Tamas. Animals cannot have any high thoughts; nor can the angels, or Devas, attain to direct freedom without human birth.

In human society, in the same way, too much wealth or too much poverty is a great impediment to the higher development of the soul. It is from the middle classes that the great ones of the world come. Here the forces are very equally adjusted and balanced.

Returning to our subject, we come next to Pranayarna, controlling the breathing. What has that to do with concentrating the powers of the mind? Breath is like the fly-wheel of this machine, the body. In a big engine you find the fly-wheel first moving, and that motion is conveyed to finer and finer machinery until the most delicate and finest mechanism in the machine is in motion. The breath is that fly-wheel, supplying and regulating the motive power to everything in this body.

There was once a minister to a great king. He fell into disgrace. The king, as a punishment, ordered him to be shut up in the top of a very high tower. This was done, and the minister was left there to perish.

He had a faithful wife, however, who came to the tower at night and called to her husband at the top to know what she could do to help him. He told her to return to the tower the following night and bring with her a long rope, some stout twine, pack thread, silken thread, a beetle, and a little honey.

Wondering much, the good wife obeyed her husband, and brought him the desired articles. The husband directed her to attach the silken thread firmly to the beetle, then to smear its horns with a drop of honey, and to set it free on the wall of the tower, with its head pointing upwards.

She obeyed all these instructions, and the beetle started on its long journey. Smelling the honey ahead it slowly crept onwards, in the hope of reaching the honey, until at last it reached the top of the tower, when the minister grasped the beetle, and got possession of the silken thread.

He told his wife to tie the other end to the pack thread, and after he had drawn up the pack thread, he repeated the process with the stout twine, and lastly with the rope. Then the rest was easy.

The minister descended from the tower by means of the rope, and made his escape.

In this body of ours the breath motion is the "silken thread"; by laying hold of and learning to control it we grasp the pack thread of the nerve currents, and from these the stout twine of our thoughts, and lastly the rope of Prana, controlling which we reach freedom.

We do not know anything about our own bodies; we cannot know. At best we can take a dead body, and cut it in pieces, and there are some who can take a live animal and cut it in pieces in order to see what is inside the body.

Still, that has nothing to do with our own bodies. We know very little about them. Why do we not? Because our attention is not discriminating enough to catch the very fine movements that are going on within. We can know of them only when the mind becomes more subtle and enters, as it were, deeper into the body.

To get the subtle perception we have to begin with the grosser perceptions. We have to get hold of that which is setting the whole engine in motion. That is the Prana, the most obvious manifestation of which is the breath.

Then, along with the breath, we shall slowly enter the body, which will enable us to find out about the subtle forces, the nerve currents that are moving all over the body. As soon as we perceive and learn to feel them, we shall begin to get control over them, and over the body.

The mind is also set in motion: by these different nerve currents, so at last we shall reach the state of perfect control over the body and the mind, making both our servants. Knowledge is power. We have to get this power.

So we must begin at the beginning, with Pranayama, restraining the Prana. This Pranayama is a long subject, and will take several lessons to illustrate it thoroughly. We shall take it part by part.

We shall gradually see the reasons for each exercise and what forces in the body are set in motion. All these things will come to us, but it requires constant practice, and the proof will come by practice. No amount of reasoning which I can give you will be proof to you, until you have demonstrated it for yourselves. As soon as you begin to feel these currents in motion all over you, doubts will vanish, but it requires hard practice every day.

You must practice at least twice every day, and the best times are towards the morning and the evening. When night passes into day, and day into night, a state of relative calmness ensues. The early morning and the early evening are the two periods of calmness. Your body will have a like tendency to become calm at those times. We should take advantage of that natural condition and begin then to practice.

Make it a rule not to eat until you have practiced; if you do this, the sheer force of hunger will break your laziness. In India they teach children never to eat until they have practiced or worshipped, and it becomes natural to them after a time; a boy will not feel hungry until he has bathed and practiced.

Those of you who can afford it will do better to have a room for this practice alone. Do not sleep in that room, it must be kept holy. You must not enter the room until you have bathed, and are perfectly clean in body and mind.

Place flowers in that room always; they are the best surroundings for a Yogi; also pictures that are pleasing. Burn incense morning and evening.

Have no quarrelling, nor anger, nor unholy thought in that room. Only allow those persons to enter it who are of the same thought as you. Then gradually there will be an atmosphere of holiness in the room, so that when you are miserable, sorrowful, doubtful, or your mind is disturbed, the very fact of entering that room will make you calm.

This was the idea of the temple and the church, and in some temples and churches you will find it even now, but in the majority of them the very idea has been lost. The idea is that by keeping holy vibrations there the place becomes and remains illumined.

Those who cannot afford to have a room set apart can practice anywhere they like. Sit in a straight posture, and the first thing to do is to send a current of holy thought to all creation.

Mentally repeat, "Let all beings be happy; let all beings be peaceful; let all beings be blissful." So do to the east, south, north and west.

The more you do that the better you will feel yourself. You will find at last that the easiest way to make ourselves healthy is to see that others are healthy, and the easiest way to make ourselves happy is to see that others are happy.

After doing that, those who believe in God should pray — not for money, not for health, nor for heaven; pray for knowledge and light; every other prayer is selfish.

Then the next thing to do is to think of your own body, and see that it is strong and healthy; it is the best instrument you have. Think of it as being as strong as adamant, and that with the help of this body you will cross the ocean of life.

Freedom is never to be reached by the weak. Throw away all weakness. Tell your body that it is strong, tell your mind that it is strong, and have unbounded faith and hope in yourself.

# More on Raja-Yoga

Yoga has essentially to do with the meditative side of religion, rather than the ethical side, though, of necessity, a little of the latter has to be considered. Men and women are growing to desire more than mere revelation, so called. They want facts in their own consciousness. Only through experience can there be any reality in religion. Spiritual facts are to be gathered mostly from the superconscious state of mind.

Let us put ourselves into the same condition as did those who claim to have had special experiences; then if we have similar experiences, they become facts for us. We can see all that another has seen; a thing that happened once can happen again, nay, must, under the same circumstances. Raja-Yoga teaches us how to reach the superconscious state.

All the great religions recognise this state in some form; but in India, special attention is paid to this side of religion. In the beginning, some mechanical means may help us to acquire this state; but mechanical means alone can never accomplish much. Certain positions, certain modes of breathing, help to harmonise and concentrate the mind, but with these must go purity and strong desire for God, or realisation. The attempt to sit down and fix the mind on one idea and hold it there will prove to most people that there is some need for help to enable them to do this successfully.

The mind has to be gradually and systematically brought under control. The will has to be strengthened by slow, continuous, and persevering drill. This is no child's play, no fad to be tried one day and discarded the next. It is a life's work; and the end to be attained is well worth all that it can cost us to reach it; being nothing less than the realisation of our absolute oneness with the Divine. Surely, with this end in view, and with the knowledge that we can certainly succeed, no price can be too great to pay.

According to Yoga philosophy, it is through ignorance that the soul has been joined with nature. The aim is to get rid of nature's control over us. That is the goal of all religions.

Each soul is potentially divine. The goal is to manifest this Divinity within, by controlling nature, external and internal. Do this either by work, or worship, or psychic control, or philosophy — by one or more or all of these — and be free. This is the whole of religion.

Doctrines, or dogmas, or rituals, or books, or temples, or forms, are but secondary details. The Yogi tries to reach this goal through psychic control. Until we can free ourselves from nature, we are slaves; as she dictates so we must go.

The Yogi claims that he who controls mind controls matter also. The internal nature is much higher than the external and much more difficult to grapple with, much more difficult to control. Therefore he who has conquered the internal nature controls the whole universe; it becomes his servant.

Raja-Yoga propounds the methods of gaining this control. Forces higher than we know in physical nature will have to be subdued. This body is just the external crust of the mind. They are not two different things; they are just as the oyster and its shell. They are but two aspects of one thing; the internal substance of the oyster takes up matter from outside, and manufactures the shell. In the same way the internal fine forces which are called mind take up gross matter from outside, and from that manufacture this external shell, the body.

If, then, we have control of the internal, it is very easy to have control of the external. Then again, these forces are not different. It is not that some forces are physical, and some mental; the physical forces are but the gross manifestations of the fine forces, just as the physical world is but the gross manifestation of the fine world.

The Yogi has a science that manufactures an instrument for the study of his own mind, and that instrument is in the mind. The mind attains to powers of finer perception which no instrument will ever be able to attain.

To attain to this power of superfine perception we have to begin from the gross. And as the power becomes finer and finer, we go deeper and deeper inside our own nature; and all the gross movements will first be tangible to us, and then the finer movements of the thought; we will be able to trace the thought before its beginning, trace it where it goes and where it ends.

For instance, in the ordinary mind a thought arises. The mind does not know how it began or whence it comes. The mind is like the ocean in which a wave rises, but although the man sees the wave, he does not know how the wave came there, whence its birth, or whither it melts down again; he cannot trace it any further.

But when the perception becomes finer, we can trace this wave long, long before it comes to the surface; and we will be able to trace it for a long distance after it has disappeared, and then we can understand psychology as it truly is.

Nowadays men think this or that and write many volumes, which are entirely misleading, because they have not the power to analyse their own minds and are talking of things they have never known , but only theorised about. All science must be based on facts, and these facts must be observed and generalised. Until you have some facts to generalise upon, what are you going to do?

So all these attempts at generalising are based upon knowing the things we generalise. A man proposes a theory, and adds theory to theory, until the whole book is patchwork of theories, not one of them with the least meaning.

The science of Râja-Yoga says, first you must gather facts about your own mind, and that can be done by analysing your mind, developing its finer powers of perception and seeing for yourselves what is happening inside; and when you have got these facts, then generalise; and then alone you will have the real science of psychology.

As I have said, to come to any finer perception we must take the help of the grosser end of it. The current of action which is manifested on the outside is the grosser. If we can get hold of this and go on further and further, it becomes finer and finer, and at last the finest.

So this body and everything we have in this body are not different existences, but, as it were, various links in the same chain proceeding from fine to gross. You are a complete whole; this body is the outside manifestation, the crust, of the inside; the external is grosser and the inside finer; and so finer and finer until you come to the Self.

And at last, when we come to the Self, we come to know that it was only the Self that was manifesting all this; that it was the Self which became the mind and became the body; that nothing else exists but the Self, and all these others are manifestations of that Self in various degrees, becoming grosser and grosser.

So we will find by analogy that in this whole universe there is the gross manifestation, and behind that is the finer movement, which we can call the will of God. Behind that even, we will find that Universal Self. And then we will come to know that the Universal Self becomes God and becomes this universe; and that it is not that this universe is one and God another and the Supreme Self another, but that they are different states of the manifestation of the same Unity behind.

The Râja-Yogi knows that the whole of nature is intended for the soul to acquire experience, and that the result of all the experiences of the soul is for it to become aware of its eternal separateness from nature. The human soul has to understand and realise that it has been spirit, and not matter, through eternity, and that this conjunction of it with matter is and can be only for a time. The Raja-Yogi learns the lesson of renunciation through his own experience of nature.

Man as Atman is really free; as man he is bound, changed by every physical condition. As man, he is a machine with an idea of freedom; but this human body is the best and the human mind the highest mind there is. When a man attains to the Atman state, he can take a body, making it to suit himself; he is above law.

This is a statement and must be proved. Each one must prove it for himself; we may satisfy ourselves, but we cannot satisfy another. Râja-Yoga is the only science of religion that can be demonstrated; and only what I myself have proved by experience, do I teach. The full ripeness of reason is intuition, but intuition cannot antagonise reason.

The mind cannot be analysed by any external machine. Supposing you could look into my brain while I am thinking, you would only see certain molecules interchanged. You could not see thought, consciousness, ideas, images. You would simply see the mass of vibrations — chemical and physical changes. From this example we see that this sort of analysis would not do.

Is there any other method by which the mind can be analysed as mind? If there is, then the real science of religion is possible. The science of Raja-Yoga claims there is such a possibility. We can all attempt it and succeed to a certain degree. There is this great difficulty: In external sciences the object is [comparatively easy to observe]. The instruments of analysis are rigid; and both are external. But in the analysis of the mind the object and the instruments of analysis are the same thing. The subject and the object become one.

External analysis will go to the brain and find physical and chemical changes. It would never succeed [in answering the questions]: What is the consciousness? What is your imagination? Where does this vast mass of ideas you have come from, and where do they go? We cannot deny them. They are facts. I never saw my own brain. I have to take for granted I have one. But man can never deny his own conscious imagination. .

The great problem is ourselves. Am I the long chain I do not see — one piece following the other in rapid succession but quite unconnected? Am I such a state of consciousness [for ever in a flux]? Or am I something more than that — a substance, an entity, what we call the soul?

In other words, has man a soul or not? Is he a bundle of states of consciousness without any connection, or is he a unified substance? That is the great controversy. If we are merely bundles of consciousness, such a question as immortality would be merely delusion. On the other hand, if there is something in me which is a unit, a substance, then of course I am immortal. The unit cannot be destroyed or broken into pieces. Only compounds can be broken up.

All religions except Buddhism believe and struggle in some way or other to reach such a substance. Buddhism denies the substance and is quite satisfied with that. It says, this business about God, the soul, immortality, and all that — do not vex yourselves with such questions.

But all the other religions of the world cling to this substance. They all believe that the soul is the substance in man in spite of all the changes, that God is the substance which is in the universe. They all believe in the immortality of the soul. These are speculations.

Who is to decide the controversy between the Buddhists and the Christians? Christianity says there is a substance that will live for ever. The Christian says, "My Bible says so." The Buddhist says, "I do not believe in your book."

The question is: Are we the substance [the soul] or this subtle matter, the changing, billowing mind? Our minds are constantly changing. Where is the substance within? We do not find it. I am now this and now that. I will believe in the substance if for a moment you can stop these changes.

Of course all the beliefs in God and heaven are little beliefs of organised religions. Any scientific religion never proposes such things.

Yoga is the science that teaches us to stop the Chitta [the mind-stuff] from getting into these changes. Suppose you succeed in leading the mind to a perfect state of Yoga. That moment you have solved the problem. You have known what you are. You have mastered all the changes.

After that you may let the mind run about, but it is not the same mind any more. It is perfectly under your control. No more like wild horses that dash you down. You have seen God.

This is no longer a matter of speculation. There is no more Mr. So-and-So, no more books or Vedas, or controversy of preachers, or anything. You have been yourself: I am the substance beyond all these changes. I am not the changes; if I were, I could not stop them. I can stop the changes, and therefore I can never be the changes. This is the proposition of the science of Yoga.

# Six Lessons on Raja-Yoga

Râja-Yoga is as much a science as any in the world. It is an analysis of the mind, a gathering of the facts of the supersensuous world and so building up the spiritual world. All the great spiritual teachers the world has known said, "I see and I know." Jesus, Paul, and Peter all claimed actual perception of the spiritual truths they taught.

This perception is obtained by Yoga.

Neither memory nor consciousness can be the limitation of existence. There is a superconscious state. Both it and the unconscious state are sensationless, but with a vast difference between them — the difference between ignorance and knowledge. Present Yoga as an appeal to reason, as a science.

Concentration of the mind is the source of all knowledge.

Yoga teaches us to make matter our slave, as it ought to be. Yoga means "yoke", "to join", that is, to join the soul of man with the supreme Soul or God.

The mind acts in and under consciousness. What we call consciousness is only one link in the infinite chain that is our nature.

This "I" of ours covers just a little consciousness and a vast amount of unconsciousness, while over it, and mostly unknown to it, is the superconscious plane.

Through faithful practice, layer after layer of the mind opens before us, and each reveals new facts to us. We see as it were new worlds created before us, new powers are put into our hands, but we must not stop by the way or allow ourselves to be dazzled by these "beads of glass" when the mine of diamonds lies before us.

God alone is our goal. Failing to reach God, we die.

Three things are necessary to the student who wishes to succeed.

First. Give up all ideas of enjoyment in this world and the next, care only for God and Truth. We are here to know truth, not for enjoyment. Leave that to brutes who enjoy as we never can. Man is a thinking being and must struggle on until he conquers death, until he sees the light. He must not spend himself in vain talking that bears no fruit. Worship of society and popular opinion is idolatry. The soul has no sex, no country, no place, no time.

Second. Intense desire to know Truth and God. Be eager for them, long for them, as a drowning man longs for breath. Want only God, take nothing else, let not "seeming" cheat you any longer. Turn from all and seek only God.

Third. The six trainings: First — Restraining the mind from going outward. Second — Restraining the senses. Third — Turning the mind inward. Fourth — Suffering everything without murmuring. Fifth — Fastening the mind to one idea. Take the subject before you and think it out; never leave it. Do not count time. Sixth — Think constantly of your real nature. Get rid of superstition. Do not hypnotise yourself into a belief in your own inferiority. Day and night tell yourself what you really are, until you realise (actually realise) your oneness with God.

Without these disciplines, no results can be gained.

We can be conscious of the Absolute, but we can never express It. The moment we try to express It, we limit It and It ceases to be Absolute.

We have to go beyond sense limit and transcend even reason, and we have the power to do this.

# FIRST LESSON

This is a lesson seeking to bring out the individuality. Each individuality must be cultivated. All will meet at the centre. "Imagination is the door to inspiration and the basis of all thought." All prophets, poets, and discoverers have had great imaginative power. The explanation of nature is in us; the stone falls outside, but gravitation is in us, not outside.

Those who stuff themselves, those who starve themselves, those who sleep too much, those who sleep too little, cannot become Yogis. Ignorance, fickleness, jealousy, laziness, and excessive attachment are the great enemies to success in Yoga practice. The three great requisites are:

First. Purity, physical and mental; all uncleanness, all that would draw the mind down, must be abandoned.

Second. Patience: At first there will be wonderful manifestations, but they will all cease. This is the hardest period, but hold fast; in the end the gain is sure if you have patience.

Third. Perseverance: Persevere through thick and thin, through health and sickness, never miss a day in practice.

The best time for practice is the junction of day and night, the calmest time in the tides of our bodies, the zero point between two states. If this cannot be done, practise upon rising and going to bed. Great personal cleanliness is necessary — a daily bath.

After bathing, sit down and hold the seat firm, that is, imagine that you sit as firm as a rock, that nothing can move you. Hold the head and shoulders and the hips in a straight line, keeping the spinal column free; all action is along it, and it must not be impaired.

Begin with your toes and think of each part of your body as perfect; picture it so in your mind, touching each part if you prefer to do so. Pass upward bit by bit until you reach the head, thinking of each as perfect, lacking nothing. Then think of the whole as perfect, an instrument given to you by God to enable you to attain Truth, the vessel in which you are to cross the ocean and reach the shores of eternal truth.

When this has been done, take a long breath through both nostrils, throw it out again, and then hold it out as long as you comfortably can. Take four such breaths, then breathe naturally and pray for illumination.

"I meditate on the glory of that being who created this universe; may he illuminate my mind." Sit and meditate on this ten or fifteen minutes.

Tell your experiences to no one but your Guru.

Talk as little as possible.

Keep your thoughts on virtue; what we think we tend to become.

Holy meditation helps to burn out all mental impurities. All who are not Yogis are slaves; bond after bond must be broken to make us free.

All can find the reality beyond. If God is true, we must feel him as a fact, and if there is a soul, we ought to be able to see it and feel it.

The only way to find if there be a soul is to be something which is not the body.

The Yogis class our organs under two chief heads: organs of sense and organs of motion, or knowledge and action.

The internal organ or mind has four aspects. First — Manas, the cogitating or thinking faculty, which is usually almost entirely wasted, because uncontrolled; properly governed, it is a wonderful power. Second — Buddhi, the will (sometimes called the intellect). Third — Ahamkâra, the self-conscious egotism (from Aham). Fourth — Chitta, the substance in and through which all the faculties act, the floor of the mind as it were; or the sea in which the various faculties are waves.

Yoga is the science by which we stop Chitta from assuming, or becoming transformed into, several faculties. As the reflection of the moon on the sea is broken or blurred by the waves, so is the reflection of the Atman, the true Self, broken by the mental waves. Only when the sea is stilled to mirror-like calmness, can the reflection of the moon be seen, and only when the "mind-stuff", the Chitta is controlled to absolute calmness, is the Self to be recognised.

The mind is not the body, though it is matter in a finer form. It is not eternally bound by the body. This is proved as we get occasionally loosened from it. We can learn to do this at will by controlling the senses.

When we can do that fully, we shall control the universe, because our world is only what the senses bring us. Freedom is the test of the higher being. Spiritual life begins when you have loosened yourself from the control of the senses. He whose senses rule him is worldly — is a slave.

If we could entirely stop our mind-stuff from breaking into waves, it would put an end to our bodies. For millions of years we have worked so hard to manufacture these bodies that in the struggle we have forgotten our real purpose in getting them, which was to become perfect. We have grown to think that body-making is the end of our efforts. This is Mâyâ. We must break this delusion and return to our original aim and realise we are not the body, it is our servant.

Learn to take the mind out and to see that it is separate from the body. We endow the body with sensation and life and then think it is alive and real. We have worn it so long that we forget that it is not identical with us. Yoga is to help us put off our body when we please and see it as our servant, our instrument, not our ruler. Controlling the mental powers is the first great aim in Yoga practices. The second is concentrating them in full force upon any subject.

You cannot be a Yogi if you talk much.

# SECOND LESSON

(These lessons are composed of notes of class talks given by Swami Vivekananda to an intimate audience in the house of Mrs. Sara C. Bull, a devoted American disciple, and were preserved by her and finally printed in 1913 for private circulation — Ed .)

This Yoga is known as the eightfold Yoga, because it is divided into eight principal parts. These are:

First — Yama. This is most important and has to govern the whole life; it has five divisions:

1st. Not injuring any being by thought, word, or deed.

2nd. Non-covetousness in thought, word, or deed.

3rd. Perfect chastity in thought, word, or deed.

4th. Perfect truthfulness in thought, word, or deed.

5th. Non-receiving of gifts.

Second — Niyama. The bodily care, bathing daily, dietary, etc.

Third — Âsana, posture. Hips, shoulders, and head must be held straight, leaving the spine free.

Fourth — Prânâyâma, restraining the breath (in order to get control of the Prâna or vital force).

Fifth — Pratyâhâra, turning the mind inward and restraining it from going outward, revolving the matter in the mind in order to understand it.

Sixth — Dhâranâ, concentration on one subject.

Seventh — Dhyâna, meditation.

Eighth — Samâdhi, illumination, the aim of all our efforts.

Yama and Niyama are for lifelong practice. As for the others, we do as the leech does, not leave one blade of grass before firmly grasping another. In other words, we have thoroughly to understand and practise one step before taking another.

The subject of this lesson is Pranayama, or controlling the Prana. In Raja-Yoga breathing enters the psychic plane and brings us to the spiritual. It is the fly-wheel of the whole bodily system.

It acts first upon the lungs, the lungs act on the heart, the heart acts upon the circulation, this in turn upon the brain, and the brain upon the mind. The will can produce an outside sensation, and the outside sensation can arouse the will.

Our wills are weak; we do not realise their power, we are so much bound up in matter. Most of our action is from outside in. Outside nature throws us off our balance, and we cannot (as we ought) throw nature off her balance. This is all wrong; the stronger power is really within.

The great saints and teachers were those who had conquered this world of thought within themselves and so spake with power. We gain control of our mind by using first the physical regulation of the breath as the silken thread. That enables us to lay hold on one power after another until the rope of concentration delivers us from the prison of the body and we are free. Reaching freedom, we can discard the means used to bring us there.

Pranayama has three parts:

1st. Puraka — inhaling.

2nd. Kumbhaka — restraining.

3rd. Rechaka — exhaling.

There are two currents passing through the brain and circulating down the sides of the spine, crossing at the base and returning to the brain. One of these currents, called the "sun" (Pingalâ), starts from the left hemisphere of the brain, crosses at the base of the brain to the right side of the spine, and recrosses at the base of the spine, like one-half of the figure eight.

The other current, the "moon" (Idâ), reverses this action and completes this figure eight. Of course, the lower part is much longer than the upper. These currents flow day and night and make deposits of the great life forces at different points, commonly known as "plexuses"; but we are rarely conscious of them. By concentration we can learn to feel them and trace them over all parts of the body. These "sun" and "moon" currents are intimately connected with breathing, and by regulating this we get control of the body.

In the Katha Upanishad the body is described as the chariot, the mind is the reins, the intellect is the charioteer, the senses are the horses, and the objects of the senses their road. The self is the rider, seated in the chariot. Unless the rider has understanding and can make the charioteer control his horses, he can never attain the goal; but the senses, like vicious steeds, will drag him where they please and may even destroy him.

These two currents are the great "check rein" in the hands of the charioteer, and he must get control of this to control the horses. We have to get the power to become moral; until we do that, we cannot control our actions.

Yoga alone enables us to carry into practice the teachings of morality. To become moral is the object of Yoga. All great teachers were Yogis and controlled every current. The Yogis arrest these currents at the base of the spine and force them through the centre of the spinal column. They then become the current of knowledge, which only exists in the Yogi.

Second Lesson in Breathing: One method is not for all. This breathing must be done with rhythmic regularity, and the easiest way is by counting; as that is purely mechanical, we repeat the sacred word "Om" a certain number of times instead.

The process of Pranayama is as follows: Close the right nostril with the thumb and then slowly inhale through the left nostril, repeating the word "Om" four times.

Then firmly close both nostrils by placing the forefinger on the left one and hold the breath in, mentally repeating "Om" eight times.

Then, removing the thumb from the right nostril, exhale slowly through that, repeating "Om" four times.

As you close the exhalation, draw in the abdomen forcibly to expel all the air from the lungs. Then slowly inhale through the right nostril, keeping the left one closed, repeating "Om" four times. Next close the right nostril with the thumb and hold the breath while repeating "Om" eight times. Then unclose the left nostril and slowly exhale, repeating "Om" four times, drawing in the abdomen as before. Repeat this whole operation twice at each sitting, that is, making four Pranayamas, two for each nostril. Before taking your seat it is well to begin with prayer.

This needs to be practised a week; then gradually increase the duration of breathing, keeping the same ratio, that is, if you repeat "Om" six times at inhalation, then do the same at exhalation and twelve times during Kumbhaka. These exercises will make us more spiritual, more pure, more holy.

Do not be led aside into any byways or seek after power. Love is the only power that stays by us and increases. He who seeks to come to God through Raja-Yoga must be strong mentally, physically, morally, and spiritually. Take every step in that light.

Of hundreds of thousands only one soul will say, "I will go beyond, and I will penetrate to God." Few can face the truth; but to accomplish anything, we must be willing to die for Truth.

# THIRD LESSON

(These lessons are composed of notes of class talks given by Swami Vivekananda to an intimate audience in the house of Mrs. Sara C. Bull, a devoted American disciple, and were preserved by her and finally printed in 1913 for private circulation — Ed .)

Kundalini: Realise the soul not as matter, but as it is. We are thinking of the soul as body, but we must separate it from sense and thought. Then alone can we know we are immortal. Change implies the duality of cause and effect, and all that changes must be mortal. This proves that the body cannot be immortal, nor can the mind, because both are constantly changing. Only the unchangeable can be immortal, because there is nothing to act upon it.

We do not become it, we are it; but we have to clear away the veil of ignorance that hides the truth from us. The body is objectified thought. The "sun" and "moon" currents bring energy to all parts of the body. The surplus energy is stored at certain points (plexuses) along the spinal column commonly known as nerve centres.

These currents are not to be found in dead bodies and can only be traced in a healthy organism.

The Yogi has an advantage; for he is able not only to feel them, but actually to see them. They are luminous in his life, and so are the great nerve centres.

There is conscious as well as unconscious action. The Yogis possess a third kind, the superconscious, which in all countries and in all ages has been the source of all religious knowledge. The superconscious state makes no mistakes, but whereas the action of the instinct would be purely mechanical, the former is beyond consciousness.

It has been called inspiration, but the Yogi says, "This faculty is in every human being, and eventually all will enjoy it."

We must give a new direction to the "sun" and "moon" currents and open for them a new passage through the centre of the spinal cord. When we succeed in bringing the currents through this passage called "Sushumnâ", up to the brain, we are for the time being separated entirely from the body.

The nerve centre at the base of the spine near the sacrum is most important. It is the seat of the generative substance of the sexual energy and is symbolised by the Yogi as a triangle containing a tiny serpent coiled up in it. This sleeping serpent is called Kundalini, and to raise this Kundalini is the whole object of Raja-Yoga.

The great sexual force, raised from animal action and sent upward to the great dynamo of the human system, the brain, and there stored up, becomes Ojas or spiritual force. All good thought, all prayer, resolves a part of that animal energy into Ojas and helps to give us spiritual power. This Ojas is the real man and in human beings alone is it possible for this storage of Ojas to be accomplished. One in whom the whole animal sex force has been transformed into Ojas is a god. He speaks with power, and his words regenerate the world.

The Yogi pictures this serpent as being slowly lifted from stage to stage until the highest, the pineal gland, is reached. No man or woman can be really spiritual until the sexual energy, the highest power possessed by man, has been converted into Ojas.

No force can be created; it can only be directed. Therefore we must learn to control the grand powers that are already in our hands and by will power make them spiritual instead of merely animal. Thus it is clearly seen that chastity is the corner-stone of all morality and of all religion. In Raja-Yoga especially, absolute chastity in thought, word, and deed is a sine qua non . The same laws apply to the married and the single. If one wastes the most potent forces of one's being, one cannot become spiritual.

All history teaches us that the great seers of all ages were either monks and ascetics or those who had given up married life; only the pure in life can see God.

Just before making the Prânâyâma, endeavour to visualise the triangle. Close your eyes and picture it vividly in your imagination. See it surrounded by flames and with the serpent coiled in the middle. When you can clearly see the Kundalini, place it in imagination at the base of the spine, and when restraining the breath in Kumbhaka, throw it forcibly down on the head of the serpent to awaken it. The more powerful the imagination, the more quickly will the real result be attained and the Kundalini be awakened. Until it does, imagine it does: try to feel the currents and try to force them through the Sushumna. This hastens their action.

# FOURTH LESSON

Before we can control the mind we must study it. We have to seize this unstable mind and drag it from its wanderings and fix it on one idea. Over and over again this must be done. By power of will we must get hold of the mind and make it stop and reflect upon the glory of God.

The easiest way to get hold of the mind is to sit quiet and let it drift where it will for a while. Hold fast to the idea, "I am the witness watching my mind drifting. The mind is not I." Then see it think as if it were a thing entirely apart from yourself. Identify yourself with God, never with matter or with the mind.

Picture the mind as a calm lake stretched before you and the thoughts that come and go as bubbles rising and breaking on its surface. Make no effort to control the thoughts, but watch them and follow them in imagination as they float away. This will gradually lessen the circles.

For the mind ranges over wide circles of thought and those circles widen out into ever-increasing circles, as in a pond when we throw a stone into it. We want to reverse the process and starting with a huge circle make it narrower until at last we can fix the mind on one point and make it stay there.

Hold to the idea, "I am not the mind, I see that I am thinking, I am watching my mind act", and each day the identification of yourself with thought and feeling will grow less, until at last you can entirely separate yourself from the mind and actually know it to be apart from yourself.

When this is done, the mind is your servant to control as you will. The first stage of being a Yogi is to go beyond the senses. When the mind is conquered, he has reached the highest stage.

Live alone as much as possible. The seat should be of comfortable height; put first a grass mat, then a skin (fur), next a silken cover.

It is better that the seat has no back and it must stand firm.

Thoughts being pictures, we should not create them. We have to exclude all thought from the mind and make it a blank; as fast as a thought comes we have to banish it. To be able to accomplish this, we must transcend matter and go beyond our body. The whole life of man is really an effort to do this.

Each soul has its own meaning: In our nature these two things are connected.

The highest ideal we have is God. Meditate on Him. We cannot know the Knower, but we are He.

Seeing evil, we are creating it. What we are, we see outside, for the world is our mirror. This little body is a little mirror we have created, but the whole universe is our body. We must think this all the time; then we shall know that we cannot die or hurt another, because he is our own. We are birthless and deathless and we ought only to love.

"This whole universe is my body; all health, all happiness is mine, because all is in the universe." Say, "I am the universe." We finally learn that all action is from us to the mirror.

Although we appear as little waves, the whole sea is at our back, and we are one with it. No wave can exist of itself.

Imagination properly employed is our greatest friend; it goes beyond reason and is the only light that takes us everywhere.

Inspiration is from within and we have to inspire ourselves by our own higher faculties.

# FIFTH LESSON

(These lessons are composed of notes of class talks given by Swami Vivekananda to an intimate audience in the house of Mrs. Sara C. Bull, a devoted American disciple, and were preserved by her and finally printed in 1913 for private circulation — Ed .)

Pratyâhâra and Dhâranâ: Krishna says, "All who seek me by whatever means will reach me", "All must reach me." Pratyahara is a gathering toward, an attempt to get hold of the mind and focus it on the desired object. The first step is to let the mind drift; watch it; see what it thinks; be only the witness. Mind is not soul or spirit. It is only matter in a finer form, and we own it and can learn to manipulate it through the nerve energies.

The body is the objective view of what we call mind (subjective). We, the Self, are beyond both body and mind; we are "Atman", the eternal, unchangeable witness. The body is crystallised thought.

When the breath is flowing through the left nostril, it is the time for rest; when through the right, for work; and when through both, the time to meditate. When we are calm and breathing equally through both nostrils, we are in the right condition for quiet meditation. It is no use trying to concentrate at first. Control of thought will come of itself.

After sufficient practice of closing the nostrils with the thumb and forefinger, we shall be able to do it by the power of will, through thought alone.

Prânâyâma is now to be slightly changed. If the student has the name of his "Ishta" (Chosen Ideal), he should use that instead of "Om" during inhalation and exhalation, and use the word "Hum" (pronounced Hoom) during Kumbhaka.

Throw the restrained breath forcibly down on the head of the Kundalini at each repetition of the word Hum and imagine that this awakens her. Identify yourself only with God. After a while thoughts will announce their coming, and we shall learn the way they begin and be aware of what we are going to think, just as on this plane we can look out and see a person coming. This stage is reached when we have learnt to separate ourselves from our minds and see ourselves as one and thought as something apart. Do not let the thoughts grasp you; stand aside, and they will die away.

Follow these holy thoughts; go with them; and when they melt away, you will find the feet of the Omnipotent God. This is the superconscious state; when the idea melts, follow it and melt with it.

Haloes are symbols of inner light and can be seen by the Yogi. Sometimes we may see a face as if surrounded by flames and in them read the character and judge without erring. We may have our Ishta come to us as a vision, and this symbol will be the one upon which we can rest easily and fully concentrate our minds.

We can imagine through all the senses, but we do so mostly through the eyes. Even imagination is half material. In other words, we cannot think without a phantasm. But since animals appear to think, yet have no words, it is probable that there is no inseparable connection between thought and images.

Try to keep up the imagination in Yoga, being careful to keep it pure and holy. We all have our peculiarities in the way of imaginative power; follow the way most natural to you; it will be the easiest.

We are the results of all reincarnations through Karma: "One lamp lighted from another", says the Buddhist — different lamps, but the same light.

Be cheerful, be brave, bathe daily, have patience, purity, and perseverance, then you will become a Yogi in truth. Never try to hurry, and if the higher powers come, remember that they are but side-paths. Do not let them tempt you from the main road; put them aside and hold fast to your only true aim-God. Seek only the Eternal, finding which we are at rest for ever; having the all, nothing is left to strive for, and we are for ever in free and perfect existence — Existence absolute, Knowledge absolute, Bliss absolute.

# SIXTH LESSON

(These lessons are composed of notes of class talks given by Swami Vivekananda to an intimate audience in the house of Mrs. Sara C. Bull, a devoted American disciple, and were preserved by her and finally printed in 1913 for private circulation — Ed .)

Sushumnâ: It is very useful to meditate on the Sushumna. You may have a vision of it come to you, and this is the best way. Then meditate for a long time on that. It is a very fine, very brilliant thread, this living passage through the spinal cord, this way of salvation through which we have to make the Kundalini rise.

In the language of the Yogi, the Sushumna has its ends in two lotuses, the lower lotus surrounding the triangle of the Kundalini and the top one in the brain surrounding the pineal gland; between these two are four other lotuses, stages on the way:

6th. Pineal Gland.

5th. Between the Eyes.

4th. Bottom of the Throat.

3rd. Level with the Heart.

2nd. Opposite the Navel.

1st. Base of Spine.

We must awaken the Kundalini, then slowly raise it from one lotus to another till the brain is reached. Each stage corresponds to a new layer of the mind.

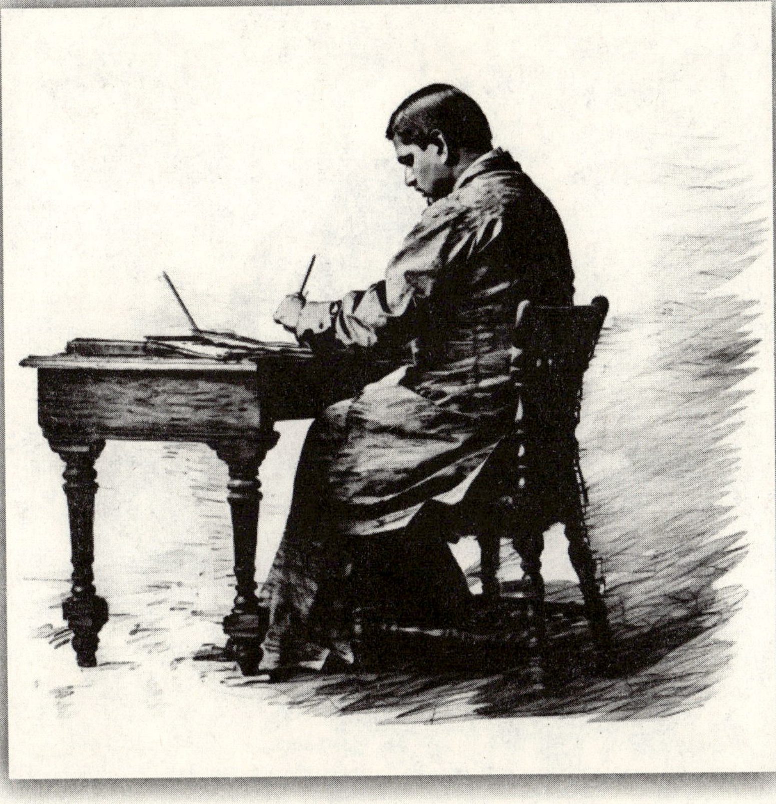

# Jnana

# First Step Towards Jnana

The word Jnâna means knowledge. It is derived from the root Jnâ — to know — the same word from which your English word to know is derived. Jnana-Yoga is Yoga by means of knowledge. What is the object of the Jnana-Yoga? Freedom. Freedom from what? Freedom from our imperfections, freedom from the misery of life. Why are we miserable? We are miserable because we are bound. What is the bondage? The bondage is of nature. Who is it that binds us? We, ourselves.

The whole universe is bound by the law of causation. There cannot be anything, any fact — either in the internal or in the external world — that is uncaused; and every cause must produce an effect.

Now this bondage in which we are is a fact. It need not be proved that we are in bondage. For instance: I would be very glad to get out of this room through this wall, but I cannot; I would be very glad if I never became sick, but I cannot prevent it; I would be very glad not to die, but I have to; I would be very glad to do millions of things that I cannot do. The will is there, but we do not succeed in accomplishing the desire. When we have any desire and not the means of fulfilling it, we get that peculiar reaction called misery. Who is the cause of desire? I, myself. Therefore, I myself am the cause of all the miseries I am in.

Misery begins with the birth of the child. Weak and helpless, he enters the world. The first sign of life is weeping. Now, how could we be the cause of misery when we find it at the very beginning? We have caused it in the past. [Here Swami Vivekananda entered into a fairly long discussion of "the very interesting theory called Reincarnation". He continued:]

To understand reincarnation, we have first to know that in this universe something can never be produced out of nothing. If there is such a thing as a human soul, it cannot be produced out of nothing. If something can be produced out of nothing, then something would disappear into nothing also. If we are produced out of nothing, then we will also go back into nothing. That which has a beginning must have an end. Therefore, as souls we could not have had any beginning. We have been existing all the time.

Then again, if we did not exist previously, there is no explanation of our present existence. The child is born with a bundle of causes. How many things we see in a child which can never be explained until we grant that the child has had past experience — for instance, fear of death and a great number of innate tendencies. Who taught the baby to drink milk and to do so in a peculiar fashion? Where did it acquire this knowledge? We know that there cannot be any knowledge without experience, for to say that knowledge is intuitive in the child, or instinctive, is what the logicians would call a "petitio principii". [299]

It would be the same [logic] as when a man asks me why light comes through a glass, and I answer him, "Because it is transparent". That would be really no answer at all because I am simply translating his word into a bigger one. The word "transparent" means "that through which light comes" — and that was the question. The question was why light comes through the glass, and I answered him, "Because it comes through the glass".

In the same way, the question was why these tendencies are in the child. Why should it have fear of death if it never saw death? If this is the first time it was ever born, how did it know to suck the mother's milk? If the answer is "Oh, it was instinct", that is simply returning the question. If a man stands up and says, "I do not know", he is in a better position than the man who says, "It is instinct" and all such nonsense.

There is no such thing as instinct; there is no such thing as nature separate from habit. Habit is one's second nature, and habit is one's first nature too. All that is in your nature is the result of habit, and habit is the result of experience. There cannot be any knowledge but from experience.

So this baby must have had some experience too. This fact is granted even by modern materialistic science. It proves beyond doubt that the baby brings with it a fund of experience. It does not enter into this world with a "tabula rasa" — a blank mind upon which nothing is written — as some of the old philosophers believed, but ready equipped with a bundle of knowledge. So far so good.

But while modern science grants that this bundle of knowledge which the child brings with it was acquired through experience, it asserts, at the same time, that it is not its own — but its father's and its grandfather's and its great-grandfather's. Knowledge comes, they say, through hereditary transmission.

Now this is one step in advance of that old theory of "instinct", that is fit only for babies and idiots. This "instinct" theory is a mere pun upon words and has no meaning whatsoever. A man with the least thinking power and the least insight into the logical precision of words would never dare to explain innate tendencies by "instinct", a term which is equivalent to saying that something came out of nothing. But the modern theory of transmission through experience — though, no doubt, a step in advance of the old one — is not sufficient at all. Why not? We can understand a physical transmission, but a mental transmission is impossible to understand.

What causes me — who am a soul — to be born with a father who has transmitted certain qualities? What makes me come back? The father, having certain qualities, may be one binding cause. Taking for granted that I am a distinct soul that was existing before and wants to reincarnate — what makes my soul go into the body of a particular man? For the explanation to be sufficient, we have to assume a hereditary transmission of energies and such a thing as my own previous experience. This is what is called Karma, or, in English, the Law of Causation, the law of fitness.

For instance, if my previous actions have all been towards drunkenness, I will naturally gravitate towards persons who are transmitting a drunkard's character. I can only take advantage of the organism produced by those parents who have been transmitting a certain peculiar influence for which I am fit by my previous actions. Thus we see that it is true that a certain hereditary experience is transmitted from father to son, and so on. At the same time, it is my past experience that joins me to the particular cause of hereditary transmission.

A simply hereditary transmission theory will only touch the physical man and would be perfectly insufficient for the internal soul of man. Even when looking upon the matter from the purest materialistic standpoint — viz. that there is no such thing as a soul in man, and man is nothing but a bundle of atoms acted upon by certain physical forces and works like an automaton — even taking that for granted, the mere transmission theory would be quite insufficient.

The greatest difficulties regarding the simple hypothesis of mere physical transmission will be here: If there be no such thing as a soul in man, if he be nothing more than a bundle of atoms acted upon by certain forces, then, in the case of transmission, the soul of the father would decrease in ratio to the number of his children; and the man who has five, six or eight children must, in the end, become an idiot. India and China — where men breed like rats — would then be full of idiots. But, on the contrary, we find that the least amount of lunacy is in India and China.

The question is, What do we mean by the word transmission ? It is a big word, but, like so many other impossible and nonsensical terms of the same kind, it has come into use without people understanding it. If I were to ask you what transmission is, you would find that you have no real conception of its meaning because there is no idea attached to it.

Let us look a little closer into the matter. Say, for instance, here is a father. A child is born to him. We see that the same qualities [which the father possesses] have entered into his child. Very good. Now how did the qualities of the father come to be in the child? Nobody knows. So this gap the modern physicists want to fill with the big word transmission . And what does this transmission mean? Nobody knows.

How can mental qualities of experience be condensed and made to live in one single cell of protoplasm? There is no difference between the protoplasm of a bird and that of a human brain. All we can say with regard to physical transmission is that it consists of the two or three protoplasmic cells cut from the father's body. That is all. But what nonsense to assume that ages and ages of past human experience got compressed into a few protoplasmic cells! It is too tremendous a pill they ask you to swallow with this little word transmission .

In olden times the churches had prestige, but today science has got it. And just as in olden times people never inquired for themselves — never studied the Bible, and so the priests had a very good opportunity to teach whatever they liked — so even now the majority of people do not study for themselves and, at the same time, have a tremendous awe and fear before anything called scientific. You ought to remember that there is a worse popery coming than ever existed in the church — the so-called scientific popery, which has become so successful that it dictates to us with more authority than religious popery.

These popes of modern science are great popes indeed, but sometimes they ask us to believe more wonderful things than any priest or any religion ever did. And one of those wonderful things is that transmission theory, which I could never understand. If I ask, "What do you mean by transmission ?" they only make it a little easier by saying, "It is hereditary transmission". And if I tell them, "That is rather Greek to me", they make it still easier by saying, "It is the adherence of paternal qualities in the protoplasmic cells". In that way it becomes easier and easier, until my mind becomes muddled and disgusted with the whole thing.

Now one thing we see: we produce thought. I am talking to you this evening and it is producing thought in your brain. By this act of transmission we understand that my thoughts are being transmitted into your brain and your mind, and producing other thoughts. This is an everyday fact.

It is always rational to take the side of things which you can understand — to take the side of fact. Transmission of thought is perfectly understandable. Therefore we are able to take up the [concept of] transmission of thought, and not of hereditary impressions of protoplasmic cells alone. We need not brush aside the theory, but the main stress must be laid upon the transmission of thought.

Now a father does not transmit thought. It is thought alone that transmits thought. The child that is born existed previously as thought. We all existed eternally as thought and will go on existing as thought.

What we think, that our body becomes. Everything is manufactured by thought, and thus we are the manufacturers of our own lives. We alone are responsible for whatever we do. It is foolish to cry out: "Why am I unhappy?" I made my own unhappiness. It is not the fault of the Lord at all.

Someone takes advantage of the light of the sun to break into your house and rob you. And then when he is caught by the policeman, he may cry: "Oh sun, why did you make me steal?" It was not the sun's fault at all, because there are thousands of other people who did much good to their fellow beings under the light of the same sun. The sun did not tell this man to go about stealing and robbing.

Each one of us reaps what we ourselves have sown. These miseries under which we suffer, these bondages under which we struggle, have been caused by ourselves, and none else in the universe is to blame. God is the least to blame for it.

"Why did God create this evil world?" He did not create this evil world at all. We have made it evil, and we have to make it good. "Why did God create me so miserable?" He did not. He gave me the same powers as [He did] to every being. I brought myself to this pass.

Is God to blame for what I myself have done? His mercy is always the same. His sun shines on the wicked and the good alike. His air, His water, His earth give the same chances to the wicked and the good. God is always the same eternal, merciful Father. The only thing for us to do is to bear the results of our own acts.

We learn that, in the first place, we have been existing eternally; in the second place that we are the makers of our own lives. There is no such thing as fate. Our lives are the result of our previous actions, our Karma. And it naturally follows that having been ourselves the makers of our Karma, we must also be able to unmake it.

The whole gist of Jnana-Yoga is to show humanity the method of undoing this Karma. A caterpillar spins a little cocoon around itself out of the substance of its own body and at last finds itself imprisoned. It may cry and weep and howl there; nobody will come to its rescue until it becomes wise and then comes out, a beautiful butterfly. So with these our bondages. We are going around and around ourselves through countless ages. And now we feel miserable and cry and lament over our bondage. But crying and weeping will be of no avail. We must set ourselves to cutting these bondages.

The main cause of all bondage is ignorance. Man is not wicked by his own nature — not at all. His nature is pure, perfectly holy. Each man is divine. Each man that you see is a God by his very nature. This nature is covered by ignorance, and it is ignorance that binds us down. Ignorance is the cause of all misery. Ignorance is the cause of all wickedness; and knowledge will make the world good. Knowledge will remove all misery. Knowledge will make us free. This is the idea of Jnana-Yoga: knowledge will make us free! What knowledge? Chemistry? Physics? Astronomy? Geology? They help us a little, just a little. But the chief knowledge is that of your own nature. "Know thyself." You must know what you are, what your real nature is. You must become conscious of that infinite nature within. Then your bondages will burst.

Studying the external alone, man begins to feel himself to be nothing. These vast powers of nature, these tremendous changes occurring — whole communities wiped off the face of the earth in a twinkling of time, one volcanic eruption shattering to pieces whole continents — perceiving and studying these things, man begins to feel himself weak. Therefore, it is not the study of external nature that makes [one] strong. But there is the internal nature of man—a million times more powerful than any volcanic eruption or any law of nature — which conquers nature, triumphs over all its laws. And that alone teaches man what he is.

"Knowledge is power", says the proverb, does it not? It is through knowledge that power comes. Man has got to know. Here is a man of infinite power and strength. He himself is by his own nature potent and omniscient. And this he must know. And the more he becomes conscious of his own Self, the more he manifests this power, and his bonds break and at last he becomes free.

How to know ourselves? the question remains now. There are various ways to know this Self, but in Jnana-Yoga it takes the help of nothing but sheer intellectual reasoning. Reason alone, intellect alone, rising to spiritual perception, shows what we are.

There is no question of believing. Disbelieve everything — that is the idea of the Jnani. Believe nothing and disbelieve everything — that is the first step. Dare to be a rationalist. Dare to follow reason wherever it leads you.

We hear everyday people saying all around us: "I dare to reason". It is, however, a very difficult thing to do. I would go two hundred miles to look at the face of the man who dares to reason and to follow reason. Nothing is easier to say, and nothing is more difficult to do. We are bound to follow superstitions all the time — old, hoary superstitions, either national or belonging to humanity in general — superstitions belonging to family, to friends, to country, to fashion, to books, to sex and to what-not.

Talk of reason! Very few people reason, indeed. You hear a man say, "Oh, I don't like to believe in anything; I don't like to grope through darkness. I must reason". And so he reasons. But when reason smashes to pieces things that he hugs unto his breast, he says, "No more! This reasoning is all right until it breaks my ideals. Stop there!" That man would never be a Jnani. That man will carry his bondage all his life and his lives to come. Again and again he will come under the power of death. Such men are not made for Jnana. There are other methods for them — such as bhakti-yoga, Karma-Yoga, or Râja-Yoga — but not Jnana-Yoga.

I want to prepare you by saying that this method can be followed only by the boldest. Do not think that the man who believes in no church or belongs to no sect, or the man who boasts of his unbelief, is a rationalist. Not at all. In modern times it is rather bravado to do anything like that.

To be a rationalist requires more than unbelief. You must be able not only to reason, but also to follow the dictates of your reason. If reason tells you that this body is an illusion, are you ready to give it up? Reason tells you that heat and cold are mere illusions of your senses; are you ready to brave these things? If reason tells you that nothing that the senses convey to your mind is true, are you ready to deny your sense perception? If you dare, you are a rationalist.

It is very hard to believe in reason and follow truth. This whole world is full either of the superstitious or of half-hearted hypocrites. I would rather side with superstition and ignorance than stand with these half-hearted hypocrites. They are no good. They stand on both sides of the river.

Take anything up, fix your ideal and follow it out boldly unto death. That is the way to salvation. Half-heartedness never led to anything. Be superstitious, be a fanatic if you please, but be something. Be something, show that you have something; but be not like these shilly-shallyers with truth — these jacks-of-all-trades who just want to get a sort of nervous titillation, a dose of opium, until this desire after the sensational becomes a habit.

The world is getting too full of such people. Contrary to the apostles who, according to Christ, were the salt of the earth, these fellows are the ashes, the dirt of the earth. So let us first clear the ground and understand what is meant by following reason, and then we will try to understand what the obstructions are to our following reason.

The first obstruction to our following reason is our unwillingness to go to truth. We want truth to come to us. In all my travels, most people told me: "Oh, that is not a comfortable religion you talk about. Give us a comfortable religion!"

I do not understand what they mean by this "comfortable religion". I was never taught any comfortable religion in my life. I want truth for my religion. Whether it be comfortable or not, I do not care. Why should truth be comfortable always? Truth many times hits hard — as we all know by our experience. Gradually, after a long intercourse with such persons, I came to find out what they meant by their stereotypical phrase. These people have got into a rut, and they do not dare to get out of it. Truth must apologize to them.

I once met a lady who was very fond of her children and her money and her everything. When I began to preach to her that the only way to God is by giving up everything, she stopped coming the next day. One day she came and told me that the reason for her staying away was because the religion I preached was very uncomfortable. "What sort of religion would be comfortable to you?" I asked in order to test her. She said: "I want to see God in my children, in my money, in my diamonds".

"Very good, madam", I replied. "You have now got all these things. And you will have to see these things millions of years yet. Then you will be bumped somewhere and come to reason. Until that time comes, you will never come to God. In the meantime, go on seeing God in your children and in your money and your diamonds and your dances."

It is difficult, almost impossible, for such people to give up sense enjoyment. It has grown upon them from birth to birth. If you ask a pig to give up his sty and to go into your most beautiful parlour, why it will be death to the pig. "Let go, I must live there", says the pig.

[Here Swami Vivekananda explained the story of the fishwife: "Once a fishwife was a guest in the house of a gardener who raised flowers. She came there with her empty basket, after selling fish in the market, and was asked to sleep in a room where flowers were kept. But, because of the fragrance of the flowers, she couldn't get to sleep for a long time. Her hostess saw her condition and said, 'Hello! Why are you tossing from side to side so restlessly?' The fishwife said: 'I don't know, friend. Perhaps the smell of the flowers has been disturbing my sleep. Can you give me my fish-basket? Perhaps that will put me to sleep'."] [300]

So with us. The majority of mankind delights in this fish smell — this world, this enjoyment of the senses, this money and wealth and chattel and wife and children. All this nonsense of the world — this fishy smell — has grown upon us. We can hear nothing beyond it, can see nothing beyond it; nothing goes beyond it. This is the whole universe.

All this talk about heaven and God and soul means nothing to an ordinary man. He has heaven already here. He has no other idea beyond this world. When you tell him of something higher, he says, "That is not a comfortable religion. Give us something comfortable". That is to say that religion is nothing but what he is doing.

If he is a thief and you tell him that stealing is the highest thing we can do, he will say, "That is a comfortable religion". If he is cheating, you have to tell him that what he is doing is all right; then he will accept your teaching as a "comfortable religion". The whole trouble is that people never want to get out of their ruts — never want to get rid of the old fish-basket and smell, in order to live. If they say, "I want the truth", that simply means that they want the fish-basket.

When have you reached knowledge? When you are equipped with

those four disciplines [i.e. the four qualifications for attainment discussed in Vedantic literature: discrimination between the real and the unreal, renunciation, the six treasures of virtue beginning with tranquillity, and longing for liberation]. You must give up all desire of enjoyment, either in this life or the next. All enjoyments of this life are vain. Let them come and go as they will.

What you have earned by your past actions none can take away from you. If you have deserved wealth, you can bury yourself in the forest and it will come to you. If you have deserved good food and clothing, you may go to the north pole and they will be brought to you. The polar bear will bring them. If you have not deserved them, you may conquer the world and will die of starvation. So, why do you bother about these things? And, after all, what is the use of them?

As children we all think that the world is made so very nice, and that masses of pleasures are simply waiting for our going out to them. That is every schoolboy's dream. And when he goes out into the world, the everyday world, very soon his dreams vanish. So with nations. When they see how every city is built upon ruins — every forest stands upon a city — then they become convinced of the vanity of this world.

All the power of knowledge and wealth once made has passed away — all the sciences of the ancients, lost, lost forever. Nobody knows how. That teaches us a grand lesson. Vanity of vanities; all is vanity and vexation of the spirit. If we have seen all this, then we become disgusted with this world and all it offers us. This is called Vairâgya, non-attachment, and is the first step towards knowledge.

The natural desire of man is to go towards the senses. Turning away from the senses takes him back to God. So the first lesson we have to learn is to turn away from the vanities of the world.

How long will you go on sinking and diving down and going up for five minutes, to again sink down, again come up and sink, and so on — tossed up and down? How long will you be whirled on this wheel of Karma — up and down, up and down? How many thousands of times have you been kings and rulers? How many times have you been surrounded by wealth and plunged into poverty? How many thousands of times have you been possessed of the greatest powers? But again you had to become men, rolling down on this mad rush of Karma's waters. This tremendous wheel of Karma stops neither for the widow's tears nor the orphan's cry.

How long will you go on? How long? Will you be like that old man who had spent all his life in prison and, when let out, begged to be brought back into his dark and filthy dungeon cell? This is the case with us all! We cling with all our might to this low, dark, filthy cell called this world — to this hideous, chimerical existence where we are kicked about like a football by every wind that blows.

We are slaves in the hands of nature — slaves to a bit of bread, slaves to praise, slaves to blame, slaves to wife, to husband, to child, slaves to everything. Why, I go about all over the world — beg, steal, rob, do anything — to make happy a boy who is, perhaps, hump-backed or ugly-looking. I will do every wicked thing to make him happy. Why? Because I am his father. And, at the same time, there are millions and millions of boys in this world dying of starvation — boys beautiful in body and in mind. But they are nothing to me. Let them all die. I am apt to kill them all to save this one rascal to whom I have given birth. This is what you call love. Not I. Not I. This is brutality.

There are millions of women — beautiful in body and mind, good, gentle, virtuous — dying of starvation this minute. I do not care for them at all. But that Jennie who is mine — who beats me three times a day, and scolds me the whole day — for that Jennie I am going to beg, borrow, cheat and steal so that she will have a nice gown.

Do you call that love? Not I. This is mere desire, animal desire — nothing more. Turn away from these things. Is there no end to these hideous dreams? Put a stop to them.

When the mind comes to that state of disgust with all the vanities of life, it is called turning away from nature. This is the first step. All desires must be given up — even the desire of getting heaven.

What are these heavens anyhow? Places where to sing psalms all the time. What for? To live there and have a nice healthy body with phosphorescent light or something of this kind coming out of every part, with a halo around the head, and with wings and the power to penetrate the wall?

If there be powers, they must pass away sooner or later. If there is a heaven — as there may be many heavens with various grades of enjoyment — there cannot be a body that lives forever. Death will overtake us, even there.

Every conjunction must have a disjunction. No body, finer or coarser, can be manufactured without particles of matter coming together. Whenever two particles come together, they are held by a certain attraction; and there will come a time when those particles will separate. This is the eternal law. So, wherever there is a body — either grosser or finer, either in heaven or on earth — death will overcome it.

Therefore, all desires of enjoyment in this life, or in a life to come, should be given up. People have a natural desire to enjoy; and when they do not find their selfish enjoyments in this life, they think that after death they will have a lot of enjoyment somewhere else. If these enjoyments do not take us towards knowledge in this life, in this world, how can they bring us knowledge in another life?

Which is the goal of man? Enjoyment or knowledge? Certainly not enjoyment. Man is not born to have pleasure or to suffer pain. Knowledge is the goal. Knowledge is the only pleasure we can have.

All the sense pleasures belong to the brute. And the more the pleasure in knowledge comes, these sense pleasures fall down. The more animal a man is, the more he enjoys the pleasures of the senses. No man can eat with the same gusto as a famished dog. No man was ever born who could feel the same pleasure in eating as an ordinary bull. See how their whole soul is in that eating. Why, your millionaires would give millions for that enjoyment in eating — but they cannot have it.

This universe is like a perfectly balanced ocean. You cannot raise a wave in one place without making a hollow in another one. The sum total of energy in the universe is the same throughout. You spend it in some place, you lose it in another. The brute has got it, but he spent it on his senses; and each of his senses is a hundred times stronger than that of man.

How the dog smells at a distance! How he traces a footstep! We cannot do that. So, in the savage man. His senses are less keen than the animal's, but keener than the civilized man's.

The lower classes in every country intensely enjoy everything physical. Their senses are stronger than those of the cultured. But as you go higher and higher in the scale, you see the power of thought increasing and the powers of the senses decreasing, in the same ratio.

Take a [brute], cut him [as it were] to pieces, and in five days he is all right. But if I scratch you, it is ten to one you will suffer for weeks or months. That energy of life which he displays — you have it too. But with you, it is used in making up your brain, in the manufacture of thought. So with all enjoyments and all pleasures. Either enjoy the pleasure of the senses — live like the brute and become a brute — or renounce these things and become free.

The great civilizations — what have they died of? They went for pleasure. And they went further down and down until, under the mercy of God, savages came to exterminate them, lest we would see human brutes growling about. Savages killed off those nations that became brutalized through sense enjoyment, lest Darwin's missing link would be found.

True civilization does not mean congregating in cities and living a foolish life, but going Godward, controlling the senses, and thus becoming the ruler in this house of the Self.

Think of the slavery in which we are [bound]. Every beautiful form I see, every sound of praise I hear, immediately attracts me; every word of blame I hear immediately repels me. Every fool has an influence over my mind. Every little movement in the world makes an impression upon me. Is this a life worth living?

So when you have realized the misery of this physical existence — when you have become convinced that such a life is not worth living — you have made the first step towards Jnana.

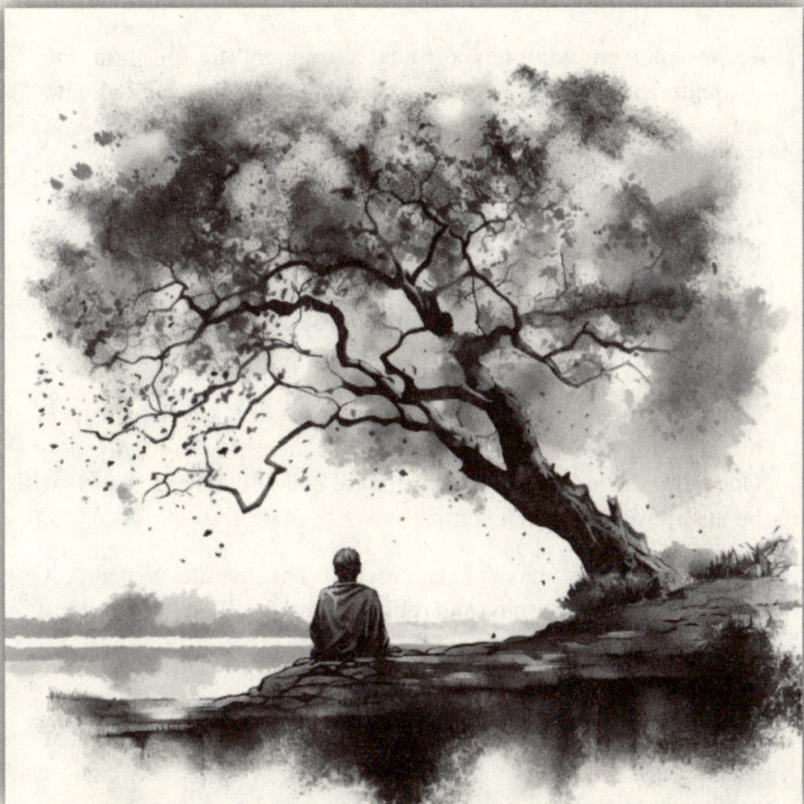

# The Real Nature of Man

Great is the tenacity with which man clings to the senses. Yet, however substantial he may think the external world in which he lives and moves, there comes a time in the lives of individuals and of races when, involuntarily, they ask, "Is this real?"

To the person who never finds a moment to question the credentials of his senses, whose every moment is occupied with some sort of sense-enjoyment — even to him death comes, and he also is compelled to ask, "Is this real?"

Religion begins with this question and ends with its answer. Even in the remote past, where recorded history cannot help us, in the mysterious light of mythology, back in the dim twilight of civilisation, we find the same question was asked, "What becomes of this? What is real?"

One of the most poetical of the Upanishads, the Katha Upanishad, begins with the inquiry: "When a man dies, there is a dispute. One party declares that he has gone for ever, the other insists that he is still living. Which is true?"

Various answers have been given. The whole sphere of metaphysics, philosophy, and religion is really filled with various answers to this question.

At the same time, attempts have been made to suppress it, to put a stop to the unrest of mind which asks, "What is beyond? What is real?"

But so long as death remains, all these attempts at suppression will always prove to be unsuccessful. We may talk about seeing nothing beyond and keeping all our hopes and aspirations confined to the present moment, and struggle hard not to think of anything beyond the world of senses; and, perhaps, everything outside helps to keep us limited within its narrow bounds.

The whole world may combine to prevent us from broadening out beyond the present. Yet, so long as there is death, the question must come again and again, "Is death the end of all these things to which we are clinging, as if they were the most real of all realities, the most substantial of all substances?"

The world vanishes in a moment and is gone. Standing on the brink of a precipice beyond which is the infinite yawning chasm, every mind, however hardened, is bound to recoil and ask, "Is this real?"

The hopes of a lifetime, built up little by little with all the energies of a great mind, vanish in a second. Are they real? This question must be answered. Time never lessens its power; on the other hand, it adds strength to it.

Then there is the desire to be happy. We run after everything to make ourselves happy; we pursue our mad career in the external world of senses. If you ask the young man with whom life is successful, he will declare that it is real; and he really thinks so.

Perhaps, when the same man grows old and finds fortune ever eluding him, he will then declare that it is fate. He finds at last that his desires cannot be fulfilled. Wherever he goes, there is an adamantine wall beyond which he cannot pass.

Every sense-activity results in a reaction. Everything is evanescent. Enjoyment, misery, luxury, wealth, power, and poverty, even life itself, are all evanescent.

Two positions remain to mankind. One is to believe with the nihilists that all is nothing, that we know nothing, that we can never know anything either about the future, the past, or even the present.

For we must remember that he who denies the past and the future and wants to stick to the present is simply a madman. One may as well deny the father and mother and assert the child. It would be equally logical. To deny the past and future, the present must inevitably be denied also.

This is one position, that of the nihilists. I have never seen a man who could really become a nihilist for one minute. It is very easy to talk.

Then there is the other position — to seek for an explanation, to seek for the real, to discover in the midst of this eternally changing and evanescent world whatever is real.

In this body which is an aggregate of molecules of matter, is there anything which is real? This has been the search throughout the history of the, human mind. In the very oldest times, we often find glimpses of light coming into men's minds.

We find man, even then, going a step beyond this body, finding something which is not this external body, although very much like it, much more complete, much more perfect, and which remains even when this body is dissolved. We read in the hymns of the Rig-Veda, addressed to the God of Fire who is burning a dead body, "Carry him, O Fire, in your arms gently, give him a perfect body, a bright body, carry him where the fathers live, where there is no more sorrow, where there is no more death."

The same idea you will find present in every religion. And we get another idea with it. It is a significant fact that all religions, without one exception, hold that man is a degeneration of what he was, whether they clothe this in mythological words, or in the clear language of philosophy, or in the beautiful expressions of poetry.

This is the one fact that comes out of every scripture and of every mythology that the man that is, is a degeneration of what he was. This is the kernel of truth within the story of Adam's fall in the Jewish scripture. This is again and again repeated in the scriptures of the Hindus; the dream of a period which they call the Age of Truth, when no man died unless he wished to die, when he could keep his body as long as he liked, and his mind was pure and strong. There was no evil and no misery; and the present age is a corruption of that state of perfection.

Side by side with this, we find the story of the deluge everywhere.

That story itself is a proof that this present age is held to be a corruption of a former age by every religion. It went on becoming more and more corrupt until the deluge swept away a large portion of mankind, and again the ascending series began. It is going up slowly again to reach once more that early state of purity.

You are all aware of the story of the deluge in the Old Testament. The same story was current among the ancient Babylonians, the Egyptians, the Chinese, and the Hindus.

Manu, a great ancient sage, was praying on the bank of the Gangâ, when a little minnow came to him for protection, and he put it into a pot of water he had before him. "What do you want?" asked Manu.

The little minnow declared he was pursued by a bigger fish and wanted protection. Manu carried the little fish to his home, and in the morning he had become as big as the pot and said, "I cannot live in this pot any longer".

Manu put him in a tank, and the next day he was as big as the tank and declared he could not live there any more. So Manu had to take him to a river, and in the morning the fish filled the river.

Then Manu put him in the ocean, and he declared, "Manu, I am the Creator of the universe. I have taken this form to come and warn you that I will deluge the world. You build an ark and in it put a pair of every kind of animal, and let your family enter the ark, and there will project out of the water my horn. Fasten the ark to it; and when the deluge subsides, come out and people the earth."

So the world was deluged, and Manu saved his own family and two of every kind of animal and seeds of every plant. When the deluge subsided, he came and peopled the world; and we are all called "man", because we are the progeny of Manu.

Now, human language is the attempt to express the truth that is within. I am fully persuaded that a baby whose language consists of unintelligible sounds is attempting to express the highest philosophy, only the baby has not the organs to express it nor the means.

The difference between the language of the highest philosophers and the utterances of babies is one of degree and not of kind. What you call the most correct, systematic, mathematical language of the present time, and the hazy, mystical, mythological languages of the ancients, differ only in degree. All of them have a grand idea behind, which is, as it were, struggling to express itself; and often behind these ancient mythologies are nuggets of truth; and often, I am sorry to say, behind the fine, polished phrases of the moderns is arrant trash.

So, we need not throw a thing overboard because it is clothed in mythology, because it does not fit in with the notions of Mr. So-and-so or Mrs. So-and-so of modern times. If people should laugh at religion because most religions declare that men must believe in mythologies taught by such and such a prophet, they ought to laugh more at these moderns.

In modern times, if a man quotes a Moses or a Buddha or a Christ, he is laughed at; but let him give the name of a Huxley, a Tyndall, or a Darwin, and it is swallowed without salt. "Huxley has said it", that is enough for many.

We are free from superstitions indeed! That was a religious superstition, and this a scientific superstition; only, in and through that superstition came life-giving ideas of spirituality; in and through this modern superstition come lust and greed. That superstition was worship of God, and this superstition is worship of filthy lucre, of fame or power. That is the difference.

To return to mythology. Behind all these stories we find one idea standing supreme — that man is a degeneration of what he was. Coming to the present times, modern research seems to repudiate this position absolutely.

Evolutionists seem to contradict entirely this assertion. According to them, man is the evolution of the mollusc; and, therefore, what mythology states cannot be true.

There is in India, however, a mythology which is able to reconcile both these positions. The Indian mythology has a theory of cycles, that all progression is in the form of waves. Every wave is attended by a fall, and that by a rise the next moment, that by a fall in the next, and again another rise. The motion is in cycles.

Certainly it is true, even on the grounds of modern research, that man cannot be simply an evolution. Every evolution presupposes an involution. The modern scientific man will tell you that you can only get the amount of energy out of a machine which you have previously put into it. Something cannot be produced out of nothing. If a man is an evolution of the mollusc, then the perfect man — the Buddha-man, the Christ-man — was involved in the mollusc.

If it is not so, whence come these gigantic personalities? Something cannot come out of nothing. Thus we are in the position of reconciling the scriptures with modern light. That energy which manifests itself slowly through various stages until it becomes the perfect man, cannot come out of nothing. It existed somewhere; and if the mollusc or the protoplasm is the first point to which you can trace it, that protoplasm, somehow or other, must have contained the energy.

There is a great discussion going on as to whether the aggregate of materials we call the body is the cause of manifestation of the force we call the soul, thought, etc., or whether it is the thought that manifests this body. The religions of the world of course hold that the force called thought manifests the body, and not the reverse. There are schools of modern thought which hold that what we call thought is simply the outcome of the adjustment of the parts of the machine which we call body.

Taking the second position that the soul or the mass of thought, or however you may call it, is the outcome of this machine, the outcome of the chemical and physical combinations of matter making up the body and brain, leaves the question unanswered.

What makes the body? What force combines the molecules into the body form? What force is there which takes up material from the mass of matter around and forms my body one way, another body another way, and so on? What makes these infinite distinctions?

To say that the force called soul is the outcome of the combinations of the molecules of the body is putting the cart before the horse. How did the combinations come; where was the force to make them? If you say that some other force was the cause of these combinations, and soul was the outcome of that matter, and that soul — which combined a certain mass of matter — was itself the result of the combinations, it is no answer.

That theory ought to be taken which explains most of the facts, if not all, and that without contradicting other existing theories. It is more logical to say that the force which takes up the matter and forms the body is the same which manifests through that body.

To say, therefore, that the thought forces manifested by the body are the outcome of the arrangement of molecules and have no independent existence has no meaning; neither can force evolve out of matter. Rather it is possible to demonstrate that what we call matter does not exist at all. It is only a certain state of force.

Solidity, hardness, or any other state of matter can be proved to be the result of motion. Increase of vortex motion imparted to fluids gives them the force of solids. A mass of air in vortex motion, as in a tornado, becomes solid-like and by its impact breaks or cuts through solids. A thread of a spider's web, if it could be moved at almost infinite velocity, would be as strong as an iron chain and would cut through an oak tree.

Looking at it in this way, it would be easier to prove that what we call matter does not exist. But the other way cannot be proved.

What is the force which manifests itself through the body? It is obvious to all of us, whatever that force be, that it is taking particles up, as it were, and manipulating forms out of them — the human body.

None else comes here to manipulate bodies for you and me.

I never saw anybody eat food for me. I have to assimilate it, manufacture blood and bones and everything out of that food. What is this mysterious force? Ideas about the future and about the past seem to be terrifying to many. To many they seem to be mere speculation.

We will take the present theme. What is this force which is now working through us? We know how in old times, in all the ancient scriptures, this power, this manifestation of power, was thought to be a bright substance having the form of this body, and which remained even after this body fell.

Later on, however, we find a higher idea coming — that this bright body did not represent the force. Whatsoever has form must be the result of combinations of particles and requires something else behind it to move it. If this body requires something which is not the body to manipulate it, the bright body, by the same necessity, will also require something other than itself to manipulate it.

So, that something was called the soul, the Atman in Sanskrit. It was the Atman which through the bright body, as it were, worked on the gross body outside. The bright body is considered as the receptacle of the mind, and the Atman is beyond that It is not the mind even; it works the mind, and through the mind the body.

You have an Atman, I have another each one of us has a separate Atman and a separate fine body, and through that we work on the gross external body.

Questions were then asked about this Atman about its nature. What is this Atman, this soul of man which is neither the body nor the mind? Great discussions followed. Speculations were made, various shades of philosophic inquiry came into existence; and I shall try to place before you some of the conclusions that have been reached about this Atman.

The different philosophies seem to agree that this Atman, whatever it be, has neither form nor shape, and that which has neither form nor shape must be omnipresent. Time begins with mind, space also is in the mind. Causation cannot stand without time. Without the idea of succession there cannot be any idea of causation.

Time, space and causation, therefore, are in the mind. And as this Atman is beyond the mind and formless, it must be beyond time, beyond space, and beyond causation.

Now, if it is beyond time, space, and causation, it must be infinite. Then comes the highest speculation in our philosophy. The infinite cannot be two. If the soul be infinite, there can be only one Soul, and all ideas of various souls — you having one soul, and I having another, and so forth — are not real.

The Real Man, therefore, is one and infinite, the omnipresent Spirit. And the apparent man is only a limitation of that Real Man. In that sense the mythologies are true that the apparent man, however great he may be, is only a dim reflection of the Real Man who is beyond.

The Real Man, the Spirit, being beyond cause and effect, not bound by time and space, must, therefore, be free. He was never bound, and could not be bound. The apparent man, the reflection, is limited by time, space, and causation, and is, therefore, bound.

Or in the language of some of our philosophers, he appears to be bound, but really is not. This is the reality in our souls, this omnipresence, this spiritual nature, this infinity. Every soul is infinite, therefore there is no question of birth and death.

Some children were being examined. The examiner put them rather hard questions, and among them was this one: "Why does not the earth fall?" He wanted to evoke answers about gravitation. Most of the children could not answer at all; a few answered that it was gravitation or something.

One bright little girl answered it by putting another question: "Where should it fall?"

The question is nonsense. Where should the earth fall? There is no falling or rising for the earth. In infinite space there is no up or down; that is only in the relative. Where is the going or coming for the infinite? Whence should it come and whither should it go?

Thus, when people cease to think of the past or future, when they give up the idea of body, because the body comes and goes and is limited, then they have risen to a higher ideal. The body is not the Real Man, neither is the mind, for the mind waxes and wanes. It is the Spirit beyond, which alone can live for ever.

The body and mind are continually changing, and are, in fact, only names of series of changeful phenomena, like rivers whose waters are in a constant state of flux, yet presenting the appearance of unbroken streams. Every particle in this body is continually changing; no one has the same body for many minutes together, and yet we think of it as the same body. So with the mind; one moment it is happy, another moment unhappy; one moment strong, another weak; an ever-changing whirlpool.

That cannot be the Spirit which is infinite. Change can only be in the limited. To say that the infinite changes in any way is absurd; it cannot be. You can move and I can move, as limited bodies; every particle in this universe is in a constant state of flux, but taking the universe as a unit, as one whole, it cannot move, it cannot change.

Motion is always a relative thing. I move in relation to something else. Any particle in this universe can change in relation to any other particle; but take the whole universe as one, and in relation to what can it move? There is nothing besides it. So this infinite Unit is unchangeable, immovable, absolute, and this is the Real Man.

Our reality, therefore, consists in the Universal and not in the limited. These are old delusions, however comfortable they are, to think that we are little limited beings, constantly changing.

People are frightened when they are told that they are Universal Being, everywhere present. Through everything you work, through every foot you move, through every lip you talk, through every heart you feel.

People are frightened when they are told this. They will again and again ask you if they are not going to keep their individuality.

What is individuality? I should like to see it. A baby has no moustache; when he grows to be a man, perhaps he has a moustache and beard. His individuality would be lost, if it were in the body. If I lose one eye, or if I lose one of my hands, my individuality would be lost if it were in the body.

Then, a drunkard should not give up drinking because he would lose his individuality. A thief should not be a good man because he would thereby lose his individuality. No man ought to change his habits for fear of this.

There is no individuality except in the Infinite. That is the only condition which does not change. Everything else is in a constant state of flux. Neither can individuality be in memory.

Suppose, on account of a blow on the head I forget all about my past; then, I have lost all individuality; I am gone. I do not remember two or three years of my childhood, and if memory and existence are one, then whatever I forget is gone. That part of my life which I do not remember, I did not live. That is a very narrow idea of individuality.

We are not individuals yet. We are struggling towards individuality, and that is the Infinite, that is the real nature of man. He alone lives whose life is in the whole universe, and the more we concentrate our lives on limited things, the faster we go towards death. Those moments alone we live when our lives are in the universe, in others; and living this little life is death, simply death, and that is why the fear of death comes.

The fear of death can only be conquered when man realises that so long as there is one life in this universe, he is living. When he can say, "I am in everything, in everybody, I am in all lives, I am the universe," then alone comes the state of fearlessness.

To talk of immortality in constantly changing things is absurd. Says an old Sanskrit philosopher: It is only the Spirit that is the individual, because it is infinite. No infinity can be divided; infinity cannot be broken into pieces. It is the same one, undivided unit for ever, and this is the individual man, the Real Man.

The apparent man is merely a struggle to express, to manifest this individuality which is beyond; and evolution is not in the Spirit. These changes which are going on — the wicked becoming good, the animal becoming man, take them in whatever way you like — are not in the Spirit. They are evolution of nature and manifestation of Spirit.

Suppose there is a screen hiding you from me, in which there is a small hole through which I can see some of the faces before me, just a few faces. Now suppose the hole begins to grow larger and larger, and as it does so, more and more of the scene before me reveals itself and when at last the whole screen has disappeared, I stand face to face with you all. You did not change at all in this case; it was the hole that was evolving, and you were gradually manifesting yourselves.

So it is with the Spirit. No perfection is going to be attained. You are already free and perfect.

What are these ideas of religion and God and searching for the hereafter? Why does man look for a God? Why does man, in every nation, in every state of society, want a perfect ideal somewhere, either in man, in God, or elsewhere?

Because that idea is within you. It was your own heart beating and you did not know; you were mistaking it for something external. It is the God within your own self that is propelling you to seek for Him, to realise Him.

After long searches here and there, in temples and in churches, in earths and in heavens, at last you come back, completing the circle from where you started, to your own soul and find that He for whom you have been seeking all over the world, for whom you have been weeping and praying in churches and temples, on whom you were looking as the mystery of all mysteries shrouded in the clouds, is nearest of the near, is your own Self, the reality of your life, body, and soul.

That is your own nature. Assert it, manifest it. Not to become pure, you are pure already. You are not to be perfect, you are that already. Nature is like that screen which is hiding the reality beyond. Every good thought that you think or act upon is simply tearing the veil, as it were; and the purity, the Infinity, the God behind, manifests Itself more and more.

This is the whole history of man. Finer and finer becomes the veil, more and more of the light behind shines forth, for it is its nature to shine. It cannot be known; in vain we try to know it. Were it knowable, it would not be what it is, for it is the eternal subject.

Knowledge is a limitation, knowledge is objectifying. He is the eternal subject of everything, the eternal witness in this universe, your own Self. Knowledge is, as it were, a lower step, a degeneration.

We are that eternal subject already; how can we know it? It is the real nature of every man, and he is struggling to express it in various ways; otherwise, why are there so many ethical codes? Where is the explanation of all ethics?

One idea stands out as the centre of all ethical systems, expressed in various forms, namely, doing good to others. The guiding motive of mankind should be charity towards men, charity towards all animals.

But these are all various expressions of that eternal truth that, "I am the universe; this universe is one." Or else, where is the reason? Why should I do good to my fellowmen? Why should I do good to others? What compels me?

It is sympathy, the feeling of sameness everywhere. The hardest hearts feel sympathy for other beings sometimes. Even the man who gets frightened if he is told that this assumed individuality is really a delusion, that it is ignoble to try to cling to this apparent individuality, that very man will tell you that extreme self-abnegation is the centre of all morality.

And what is perfect self-abnegation? It means the abnegation of this apparent self, the abnegation of all selfishness. This idea of "me and mine" — Ahamkâra and Mamatâ — is the result of past Superstition, and the more this present self passes away, the more the real Self becomes manifest.

This is true self-abnegation, the centre, the basis, the gist of all moral teaching; and whether man knows it or not the whole world is slowly going towards it, practicing it more or less. Only, the vast majority of mankind are doing it unconsciously.

Let them do it consciously. Let them make the sacrifice, knowing that this "me and mine" is not the real Self, but only a limitation. But one glimpse Of that infinite reality which is behind — but one spark of that infinite fire that is the All — represents the present man; the Infinite is his true nature.

What is the utility, the effect, the result, of this knowledge? In these days, we have to measure everything by utility — by how many pounds shillings, and pence it represents.

What right has a person to ask that truth should be judged by the standard of utility or money? Suppose there is no utility, will it be less true? Utility is not the test of truth.

Nevertheless, there is the highest utility in this. Happiness, we see is what everyone is seeking for, but the majority seek it in things which are evanescent and not real.

No happiness was ever found in the senses. There never was a person who found happiness in the senses or in enjoyment of the senses. Happiness is only found in the Spirit. Therefore the highest utility for mankind is to find this happiness in the Spirit.

The next point is that ignorance is the great mother of all misery, and the fundamental ignorance is to think that the Infinite weeps and cries, that He is finite. This is the basis of all ignorance that we, the immortal, the ever pure, the perfect Spirit, think that we are little minds, that we are little bodies; it is the mother of all selfishness.

As soon as I think that I am a little body, I want to preserve it, to protect it, to keep it nice, at the expense of other bodies; then you and I become separate. As soon as this idea of separation comes, it opens the door to all mischief and leads to all misery. This is the utility that if a very small fractional part of human beings living today can put aside the idea of selfishness, narrowness, and littleness, this earth will become a paradise tomorrow.

But with machines and improvements of material knowledge only, it will never be. These only increase misery, as oil poured on fire increases the flame all the more. Without the knowledge of the Spirit, all material knowledge is only adding fuel to fire, only giving into the hands of selfish man one more instrument to take what belongs to others, to live upon the life of others, instead of giving up his life for them.

Is it practical? — is another question. Can it be practised in modern society? Truth does not pay homage to any society, ancient or modern. Society has to pay homage to Truth or die. Societies should be moulded upon truth, and truth has not to adjust itself to society. If such a noble truth as unselfishness cannot be practiced in society, it is better for man to give up society and go into the forest.

That is the daring man. There are two sorts of courage. One is the courage of facing the cannon. And the other is the courage of spiritual conviction.

An Emperor who invaded India was told by his teacher to go and see some of the sages there. After a long search for one, he found a very old man sitting on a block of stone.

The Emperor talked with him a little and became very much impressed by his wisdom. He asked the sage to go to his country with him.

"No," said the sage, "I am quite satisfied with my forest here."

Said the Emperor, "I will give you money, position, wealth. I am the Emperor of the world."

"No," replied the man, "I don't care for those things."

The Emperor replied, "If you do not go, I will kill you."

The man smiled serenely and said, "That is the most foolish thing you ever said, Emperor. You cannot kill me. Me the sun cannot dry, fire cannot burn, sword cannot kill, for I am the birthless, the deathless, the ever-living omnipotent, omnipresent Spirit."

This is spiritual boldness, while the other is the courage of a lion or a tiger.

In the Mutiny of 1857 there was a Swami, a very great soul, whom a Mohammedan mutineer stabbed severely. The Hindu mutineers caught and brought the man to the Swami, offering to kill him.

But the Swami looked up calmly and said, "My brother, thou art He, thou art He!" and expired.

This is another instance. What good is it to talk of the strength of your muscles, of the superiority of your Western institutions, if you cannot make Truth square with your society, if you cannot build up a society into which the highest Truth will fit? What is the good of this boastful talk about your grandeur and greatness, if you stand up and say, "This courage is not practical."

Is nothing practical but pounds, shillings, and pence? If so, why boast of your society? That society is the greatest, where the highest truths become practical . That is my opinion; and if society is; not fit for the highest truths, make it so; and the sooner, the better.

Stand up, men and women, in this spirit, dare to believe in the Truth, dare to practice the Truth! The world requires a few hundred bold men and women. Practise that boldness which dares know the Truth, which dares show the Truth in life, which does not quake before death, nay, welcomes death, makes a man know that he, is the Spirit, that, in the whole universe, nothing can kill him. Then you will be free. Then you will know yours real Soul.

"This Atman is first to be heard, then thoughts about and then meditated upon."

There is a great tendency in modern times to talk too much of work and decry thought. Doing is very good, but that comes from thinking. Little manifestations of energy through the muscles are called work. But where there is no thought, there will be no work.

Fill the brain, therefore, with high thoughts, highest ideals, place them day and night before you, and out of that will come great work. Talk not about impurity, but say that we are pure. We have hypnotised ourselves into this thought that we are little, that we are born, and that we are going to die, and into a constant state of fear.

There is a story about a lioness, who was big with young, going about in search of prey; and seeing a flock of sheep, she jumped upon them. She died in the effort; and a little baby lion was born, motherless.

It was taken care of by the sheep and the sheep brought it up, and it grew up with them, ate grass, and bleated like the sheep. And although in time it became a big, full-grown lion. it thought it was a sheep.

One day another lion came in search of prey and was astonished to find that in the midst of this flock of sheep was a lion, fleeing like the sheep at the approach of danger. He tried to get near the sheep-lion, to tell it that it was not a sheep but a lion; but the poor animal fled at his approach.

However, he watched his opportunity and one day found the sheep-lion sleeping. He approached it and said, "You are a lion."

"I am a sheep," cried the other lion and could not believe the contrary but bleated.

The lion dragged him towards a lake and said, "Look here, here is my reflection and yours."

Then came the comparison. It looked at the lion and then at its own reflection, and in a moment came the idea that it was a lion. The lion roared, the bleating was gone.

You are lions, you are souls, pure, infinite, and perfect. The might of the universe is within you. "Why weepest thou, my friend? There is neither birth nor death for thee. Why weepest thou? There is no disease nor misery for thee, but thou art like the infinite sky; clouds of various colours come over it, play for a moment, then vanish. But the sky is ever the same eternal blue."

Why do we see wickedness? There was a stump of a tree, and in the dark, a thief came that way and said, "That is a policeman." A young man waiting for his beloved saw it and thought that it was his sweetheart. A child who had been told ghost stories took it for a ghost and began to shriek. But all the time it was the stump of a tree.

We see the world as we are. Suppose there is a baby in a room with a bag of gold on the table and a thief comes and steals the gold. Would the baby know it was stolen? That which we have inside, we see outside. The baby has no thief inside and sees no thief outside.

So with all knowledge. Do not talk of the wickedness of the world and all its sins. Weep that you are bound to see wickedness yet. Weep that you are bound to see sin everywhere, and if you want to help the world, do not condemn it. Do not weaken it more.

For what is sin and what is misery, and what are all these, but the results of weakness? The world is made weaker and weaker every day by such teachings.

Men are taught from childhood that they are weak and sinners. Teach them that they are all glorious children of immortality, even those who are the weakest in manifestation. Let positive, strong, helpful thought enter into their brains from very childhood. Lay yourselves open to these thoughts, and not to weakening and paralysing ones.

Say to your own minds, "I am He, I am He." Let it ring day and night in your minds like a song, and at the point of death declare "I am He." That is the Truth; the infinite strength of the world is yours.

Drive out the superstition that has covered your minds. Let us be brave. Know the Truth and practice the Truth. The goal may be distant, but awake, arise, and stop not till the goal is reached.

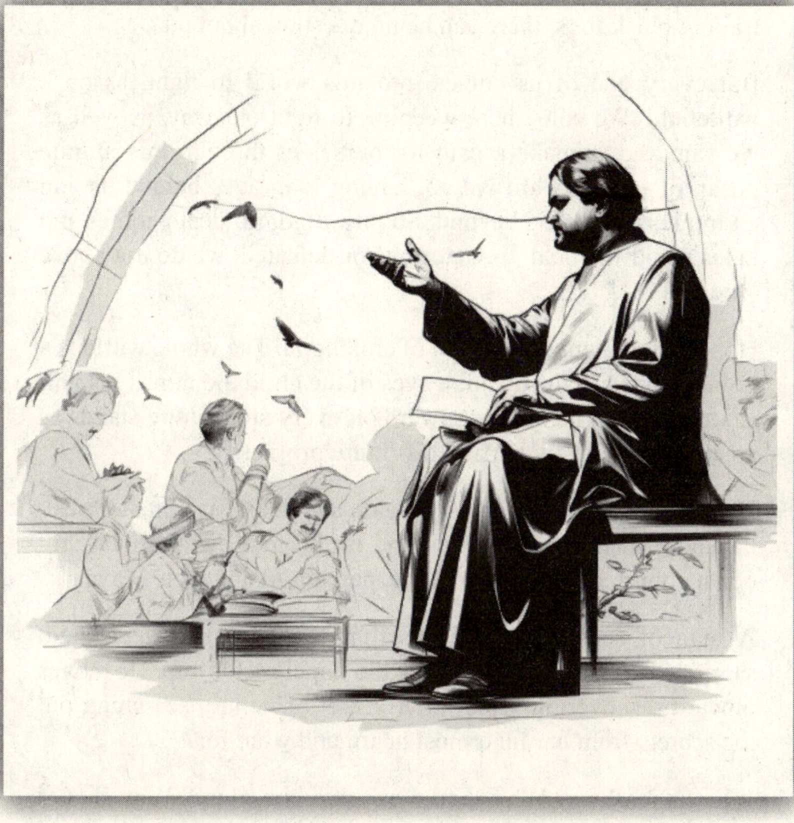

# Maya And Freedom

(Delivered in London, 22nd October 1896)

"Trailing clouds of glory we come," says the poet. Not all of us come as trailing clouds of glory however; some of us come as trailing black fogs; there can be no question about that.

But every one of us comes into this world to fight, as on a battlefield. We come here weeping to fight our way, as well as we can, and to make a path for ourselves through this infinite ocean of life; forward we go, having long ages behind us and an immense expanse beyond. So on we go, till death comes and takes us off the field — victorious or defeated, we do not know. And this is Mâyâ.

Hope is dominant in the heart of childhood. The whole world is a golden vision to the opening eyes of the child; he thinks his will is supreme. As he moves onward, at every step nature stands as an adamantine wall, barring his future progress.

He may hurl himself against it again and again, striving to break through. The further he goes, the further recedes the ideal, till death comes, and there is release, perhaps. And this is Maya.

A man of science rises, he is thirsting after knowledge. No sacrifice is too great, no struggle too hopeless for him. He moves onward discovering secret after secret of nature, searching out the secrets from her innermost heart, and what for?

What is it all for? Why should we give him glory? Why should he acquire fame? Does not nature do infinitely more than any human being can do? — and nature is dull, insentient. Why should it be glory to imitate the dull, the insentient?

Nature can hurl a thunderbolt of any magnitude to any distance. If a man can do one small part as much, we praise him and laud him to the skies. Why? Why should we praise him for imitating nature, imitating death, imitating dullness imitating insentience?

The force of gravitation can pull to pieces the biggest mass that ever existed; yet it is insentient. What glory is there in imitating the insentient? Yet we are all struggling after that. And this is maya.

The senses drag the human soul out. Man is seeking for pleasure and for happiness where it can never be found. For countless ages we are all taught that this is futile and vain, there is no happiness here. But we cannot learn; it is impossible for us to do so, except through our own experiences. We try them, and a blow comes.

Do we learn then? Not even then. Like moths hurling themselves against the flame, we are hurling ourselves again and again into sense-pleasures, hoping to find satisfaction there. We return again and again with freshened energy; thus we go on, till crippled and cheated we die. And this is Maya.

So with our intellect. In our desire to solve the mysteries of the universe, we cannot stop our questioning, we feel we must know and cannot believe that no knowledge is to be gained.

A few steps, and there arises the wall of beginningless and endless time which we cannot surmount. A few steps, and there appears a wall of boundless space which cannot be surmounted, and the whole is irrevocably bound in by the walls of cause and effect. We cannot go beyond them. Yet we struggle, and still have to struggle. And this is Maya.

With every breath, with every pulsation of the heart with every one of our movements, we think we are free, and the very same moment we are shown that we are not. Bound slaves, nature's bond-slaves, in body, in mind, in all our thoughts, in all our feelings. And this is Maya.

There was never a mother who did not think her child was a born genius, the most extraordinary child that was ever born; she dotes upon her child. Her whole soul is in the child.

The child grows up, perhaps becomes a drunkard, a brute, ill-treats the mother, and the more he ill-treats her, the more her love increases. The world lauds it as the unselfish love of the mother, little dreaming that the mother is a born slave, she cannot help it. She would a thousand times rather throw off the burden, but she cannot.

So she covers it with a mass of flowers, which she calls wonderful love. And this is Maya.

We are all like this in the world. A legend tells how once Nârada said to Krishna, "Lord, show me Maya."

A few days passed away, and Krishna asked Narada to make a trip with him towards a desert, and after walking for several miles, Krishna said, "Narada, I am thirsty; can you fetch some water for me?" "I will go at once, sir, and get you water."

So Narada went. At a little distance there was a village; he entered the village in search of water and knocked at a door, which was opened by a most beautiful young girl.

At the sight of her he immediately forgot that his Master was waiting for water, perhaps dying for the want of it. He forgot everything and began to talk with the girl. All that day he did not return to his Master.

The next day, he was again at the house, talking to the girl. That talk ripened into love; he asked the father for the daughter, and they were married and lived there and had children.

Thus twelve years passed. His father-in-law died, he inherited his property. He lived, as he seemed to think, a very happy life with his wife and children, his fields and his cattle. and so forth.

Then came a flood. One night the river rose until it overflowed its banks and flooded the whole village. Houses fell, men and animals were swept away and drowned, and everything was floating in the rush of the stream.

Narada had to escape. With one hand be held his wife, and with the other two of his children; another child was on his shoulders, and he was trying to ford this tremendous flood.

After a few steps he found the current was too strong, and the child on his shoulders fell and was borne away. A cry of despair came from Narada. In trying to save that child, he lost his grasp upon one of the others, and it also was lost. At last his wife, whom he clasped with all his might, was torn away by the current, and he was thrown on the bank, weeping and wailing in bitter lamentation.

Behind him there came a gentle voice, "My child, where is the water? You went to fetch a pitcher of water, and I am waiting for you; you have been gone for quite half an hour."

"Half an hour! " Narada exclaimed. Twelve whole years had passed through his mind, and all these scenes had happened in half an hour! And this is Maya.

In one form or another, we are all in it. It is a most difficult and intricate state of things to understand. It has been preached in every country, taught everywhere, but only believed in by a few, because until we get the experiences ourselves we cannot believe in it.

What does it show? Something very terrible. For it is all futile. Time, the avenger of everything, comes, and nothing is left. He swallows up the saint and the sinner, the king and the peasant, the beautiful and the ugly; he leaves nothing.

Everything is rushing towards that one goal, destruction. Our knowledge, our arts, our sciences, everything is rushing towards it. None can stem the tide, none can hold it back for a minute. We may try to forget it, in the same way that persons in a plague-striker city try to create oblivion by drinking, dancing, and other vain attempts, and so becoming paralysed. So we are trying to forget, trying to create oblivion by all sorts of sense-pleasures. And this is Maya.

Two ways have been proposed. One method, which everyone knows, is very common, and that is: "It may be very true, but do not think of it. 'Make hay while the sun shines,' as the proverb says. It is all true, it is a fact, but do not mind it. Seize the few pleasures you can, do what little you can, do not look at the dark side of the picture, but always towards the hopeful, the positive side."

There is some truth in this, but there is also a danger. The truth is that it is a good motive power. Hope and a positive ideal are very good motive powers for our lives, but there is a certain danger in them. The danger lies in our giving up the struggle in despair.

Such is the case with those who preach, "Take the world as it is, sit down as calmly and comfortably as you can and be contented with all these miseries. When you receive blows, say they are not blows but flowers; and when you are driven about like slaves, say that you are free. Day and night tell lies to others and to your own souls, because that is the only way to live happily."

This is what is called practical wisdom, and never was it more prevalent in the world than in this nineteenth century; because never were harder blows hit than at the present time, never was competition keener, never were men so cruel to their fellow-men as now; and, therefore, must this consolation be offered. It is put forward in the strongest way at the present time; but it fails, as it always must fail.

We cannot hide a carrion with roses; it is impossible. It would not avail long; for soon the roses would fade, and the carrion would be worse than ever before. So with our lives. We may try to cover our old and festering sores with cloth of gold, but there comes a day when the cloth of gold is removed, and the sore in all its ugliness is revealed.

Is there no hope then? True it is that we are all slaves of Maya, born in Maya, and live in Maya. Is there then no way out, no hope? That we are all miserable, that this world is really a prison, that even our so-called trailing beauty is but a prison-house, and that even our intellects and minds are prison-houses, have been known for ages upon ages.

There has never been a man, there has never been a human soul, who has not felt this sometime or other, however he may talk. And the old people feel it most, because in them is the accumulated experience of a whole life, because they cannot be easily cheated by the lies of nature.

Is there no way out? We find that with all this, with this terrible fact before us, in the midst of sorrow and suffering, even in this world where life and death are synonymous, even here, there is a still small voice that is ringing through all ages, through every country, and in every heart: "This My Maya is divine, made up of qualities, and very difficult to cross. Yet those that come unto Me, cross the river of life."

"Come unto Me all ye that labour and are heavy laden and I will give you rest."

This is the voice that is leading us forward. Man has heard it, and is hearing it all through the ages. This voice comes to men when everything seems to be lost and hope has fled, when man's dependence on his own strength has been crushed down and everything seems to melt away between his fingers, and life is a hopeless ruin. Then he hears it. This is called religion.

On the one side, therefore, is the bold assertion that this is all nonsense, that this is Maya, but along with it there is the most hopeful assertion that beyond Maya, there is a way out.

On the other hand, practical men tell us, "Don't bother your heads about such nonsense as religion and metaphysics. Live here; this is a very bad world indeed, but make the best of it."

Which put in plain language means, live a hypocritical, lying life, a life of continuous fraud, covering all sores in the best way you can. Go on putting patch after patch, until everything is lost, and you are a mass of patchwork. This is what is called practical life.

Those that are satisfied with this patchwork will never come to religion. Religion begins with a tremendous dissatisfaction with the present state of things, with our lives, and a hatred, an intense hatred, for this patching up of life, an unbounded disgust for fraud and lies.

He alone can be religious who dares say, as the mighty Buddha once said under the Bo-tree, when this idea of practicality appeared before him and he saw that it was nonsense, and yet could not find a way out. When the temptation came to him to give up his search after truth, to go back to the world and live the old life of fraud, calling things by wrong names, telling lies to oneself and to everybody, he, the giant, conquered it and said, "Death is better than a vegetating ignorant life; it is better to die on the battle-field than to live a life of defeat."

This is the basis of religion. When a man takes this stand, he is on the way to find the truth, he is on the way to God. That determination must be the first impulse towards becoming religious. I will hew out a way for myself. I will know the truth or give up my life in the attempt.

For on this side it is nothing, it is gone, it is vanishing every day. The beautiful, hopeful, young person of today is the veteran of tomorrow. Hopes and joys and pleasures will die like blossoms with tomorrow's frost. That is one side; on the other, there are the great charms of conquest, victories over all the ills of life, victory over life itself, the conquest of the universe. On that side men can stand.

Those who dare, therefore, to struggle for victory, for truth, for religion, are in the right way; and that is what the Vedas preach: Be not in despair, the way is very difficult, like walking on the edge of a razor; yet despair not, arise, awake, and find the ideal, the goal.

Now all these various manifestations of religion, in whatever shape and form they have come to mankind, have this one common central basis. It is the preaching of freedom, the way out of this world. They never came to reconcile the world and religion, but to cut the Gordian knot, to establish religion in its own ideal, and not to compromise with the world.

That is what every religion preaches, and the duty of the Vedanta is to harmonise all these aspirations, to make manifest the common ground between all the religions of the world, the highest as well as the lowest. What we call the most arrant superstition and the highest philosophy really have a common aim in that they both try to show the way out of the same difficulty, and in most cases this way is through the help of someone who is not himself bound by the laws of nature in one word, someone who is free.

In spite of all the difficulties and differences of opinion about the nature of the one free agent, whether he is a Personal God, or a sentient being like man, whether masculine, feminine, or neuter — and the discussions have been endless — the fundamental idea is the same. In spite of the almost hopeless contradictions of the different systems, we find the golden thread of unity running through them all, and in this philosophy, this golden thread has been traced revealed little by little to our view, and the first step to this revelation is the common ground that all are advancing towards freedom.

One curious fact present in the midst of all our joys and sorrows, difficulties and struggles, is that we are surely journeying towards freedom. The question was practically this: "What is this universe? From what does it arise? Into what does it go?"

And the answer was: "In freedom it rises, in freedom it rests, and into freedom it melts away."

This idea of freedom you cannot relinquish. Your actions, your very lives will be lost without it. Every moment nature is proving us to be slaves and not free. Yet, simultaneously rises the other idea, that still we are free. At every step we are knocked down, as it were, by Maya, and shown that we are bound; and yet at the same moment, together with this blow, together with this feeling that we are bound, comes the other feeling that we are free.

Some inner voice tells us that we are free. But if we attempt to realise that freedom, to make it manifest, we find the difficulties almost insuperable Yet, in spite of that it insists on asserting itself inwardly, "I am free, I am free."

And if you study all the various religions of the world you will find this idea expressed. Not only religion — you must not take this word in its narrow sense — but the whole life of society is the assertion of that one principle of freedom.

All movements are the assertion of that one freedom. That voice has been heard by everyone, whether he knows it or not, that voice which declares, "Come unto Me all ye that labour and are heavy laden."

It may not be in the same language or the same form of speech, but in some form or other, that voice calling for freedom has been with us. Yes, we are born here on account of that voice; every one of our movements is for that. We are all rushing towards freedom, we are all following that voice, whether we know it or not; as the children of the village were attracted by the music of the flute-player, so we are all following the music of the voice without knowing it.

We are ethical when we follow that voice. Not only the human soul, but all creatures, from the lowest to the highest have heard the voice and are rushing towards it; and in the struggle are either combining with each other or pushing each other out of the way.

Thus come competition, joys, struggles, life, pleasure, and death, and the whole universe is nothing but the result of this mad struggle to reach the voice. This is the manifestation of nature.

What happens then? The scene begins to shift. As soon as you know the voice and understand what it is, the whole scene changes. The same world which was the ghastly battle-field of Maya is now changed into something good and beautiful.

We no longer curse nature, nor say that the world is horrible and that it is all vain; we need no longer weep and wail. As soon as we understand the voice, we see the reassert why this struggle should be here, this fight, this competition, this difficulty, this cruelty, these little pleasures and joys; we see that they are in the nature of things, because without them there would be no going towards the voice, to attain which we are destined, whether we know it or not.

All human life, all nature, therefore, is struggling to attain to freedom. The sun is moving towards the goal, so is the earth in circling round the sun, so is the moon in circling round the earth. To that goal the planet is moving, and the air is blowing.

Everything is struggling towards that. The saint is going towards that voice — he cannot help it, it is no glory to him. So is the sinner. The charitable man is going straight towards that voice, and cannot be hindered; the miser is also going towards the same destination: the greatest worker of good hears the same voice within, and he cannot resist it, he must go towards the voice; so with the most arrant idler.

One stumbles more than another, and him who stumbles more we call bad, him who stumbles less we call good. Good and bad are never two different things, they are one and the same; the difference is not one of kind, but of degree.

Now, if the manifestation of this power of freedom is really governing the whole universe — applying that to religion, our special study — we find this idea has been the one assertion throughout.

Take the lowest form of religion where there is the worship of departed ancestors or certain powerful and cruel gods. What is the prominent idea about the gods or departed ancestors? That they are superior to nature, not bound by its restrictions.

The worshipper has, no doubt, very limited ideas of nature. He himself cannot pass through a wall, nor fly up into the skies, but the gods whom he worships can do these things. What is meant by that, philosophically? That the assertion of freedom is there, that the gods whom he worships are superior to nature as he knows it.

So with those who worship still higher beings. As the idea of nature expands, the idea of the soul which is superior to nature also expands, until we come to what we call monotheism, which holds that there is Maya (nature), and that there is some Being who is the Ruler of this Maya.

Here Vedanta begins, where these monotheistic ideas first appear. But the Vedanta philosophy wants further explanation.

This explanation — that there is a Being beyond all these manifestations of Maya, who is superior to and independent of Maya, and who is attracting us towards Himself, and that we are all going towards Him — is very good, says the Vedanta, but yet the perception is not clear, the vision is dim and hazy, although it does not directly contradict reason.

Just as in your hymn it is said, "Nearer my God to Thee," the same hymn would be very good to the Vedantin, only he would change a word, and make it, "Nearer my God to me."

The idea that the goal is far off, far beyond nature, attracting us all towards it, has to be brought nearer and nearer, without degrading or degenerating it. The God of heaven becomes the God in nature, and the God in nature becomes the God who is nature, and the God who is nature becomes the God within this temple of the body, and the God dwelling in the temple of the body at last becomes the temple itself, becomes the soul and man — and there it reaches the last words it can teach.

He whom the sages have been seeking in all these places is in our own hearts; the voice that you heard was right, says the Vedanta, but the direction you gave to the voice was wrong. That ideal of freedom that you perceived was correct, but you projected it outside yourself, and that was your mistake. Bring it nearer and nearer, until you find that it was all the time within you, it was the Self of your own self.

That freedom was your own nature, and this Maya never bound you. Nature never has power over you. Like a frightened child you were dreaming that it was throttling you, and the release from this fear is the goal: not only to see it intellectually, but to perceive it, actualise it, much more definitely than we perceive this world.

Then we shall know that we are free. Then, and then alone, will all difficulties vanish, then will all the perplexities of heart be smoothed away, all crookedness made straight, then will vanish the delusion of manifoldness and nature; and Maya instead of being a horrible, hopeless dream, as it is now will become beautiful, and this earth, instead of being a prison-house, will become our playground, and even dangers and difficulties, even all sufferings, will become deified and show us their real nature, will show us that behind everything, as the substance of everything, He is standing, and that He is the one real Self.

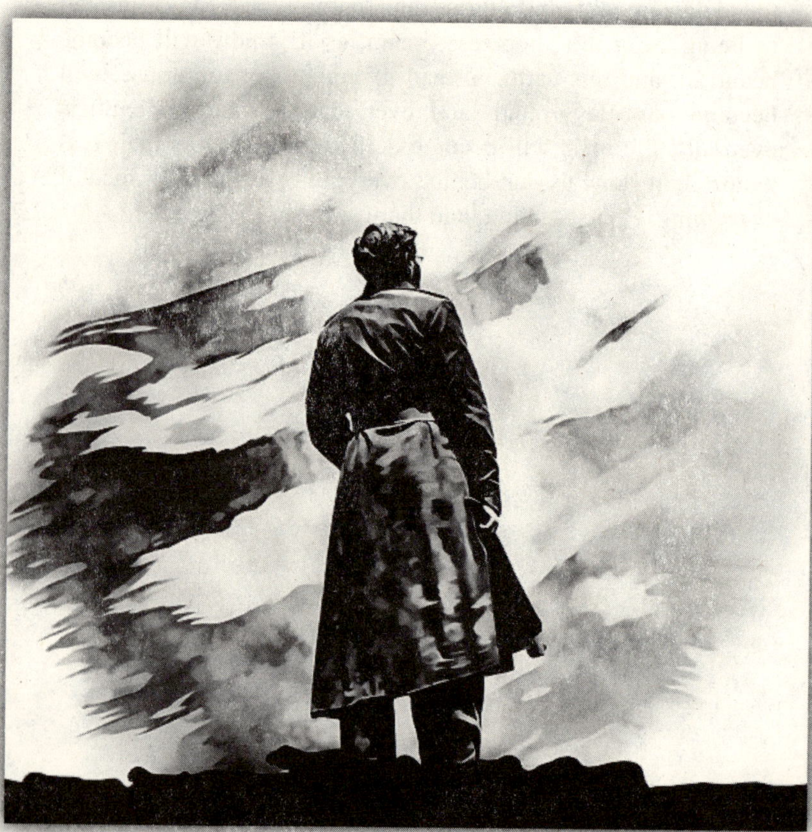

# Jnana-Yoga

Wisdom (Jnâna) is the goal of all life. We find that man enjoys his intellect more than an animal enjoys its senses; and we see that man enjoys his spiritual nature even more than his rational nature. So the highest wisdom must be this spiritual knowledge. With this knowledge will come bliss. All these things of this world are but the shadows, the manifestations in the third or fourth degree of the real Knowledge and Bliss.

This illusion of the universe will break one day. The whole of this will vanish, melt away. This is realization.

Philosophy is no joke or talk. It has to be realised; this body will vanish, this earth and everything will vanish, this idea that I am the body or the mind will for some time vanish, or if the Karma is ended it will disappear, never to come back; but if one part of the Karma remains, then as a potter's wheel, after the potter has finished the pot, will sometimes go on from the past momentum, so this body, when the delusion has vanished altogether, will go on for some time.

Again this world will come, men and women and animals will come, just as the mirage came the next day, but not with the same force; along with it will come the idea that I know its nature now, and it will cause no bondage, no more pain, nor grief, nor misery. Whenever anything miserable will come, the mind will be able to say, "I know you as hallucination."

When a man has reached that state, he is called Jivanmukta, living-free", free even while living. The aim and end in this life for the Jnâna-Yogi is to become this Jivanmukta, "living-free". He is Jivanmukta who can live in this world without being attached.

He is like the lotus leaves in water, which are never wetted by the water. He is the highest of human beings, nay, the highest of all beings, for he has realised his identity with the Absolute, he has realised that he is one with God.

If we have known the Âtman as It is, if we have known that there is nothing else but this Atman, that everything else is but a dream, with no existence in reality, then this world with its poverties, its miseries, its wickedness, and its goodness will cease to disturb us.

If they do not exist, for whom and for what shall we take trouble? This is what the Jnana-Yogis teach. Therefore, dare to be free, dare to go as far as your thought leads, and dare to carry that out in your life.

It is very hard to come to Jnâna. It is for the bravest and most daring, who dare to smash all idols, not only intellectual, but in the senses. This body is not I; it must go. All sorts of curious things may come out of this.

Who are fit to become Jnana-Yogis? Those who are equipped with these requisites: First, renunciation of all fruits of work and of all enjoyments in this life or another life. If you are the creator of this universe, whatever you desire you will have, because you will create it for yourself.

It is only a question of time. Some get it immediately; with others the past Samskâras (impressions) stand in the way of getting their desires. We give the first place to desires for enjoyment, either in this or another life.

Deny that there is any life at all; because life is only another name for death. Deny that you are a living being. Who cares for life? Life is one of these hallucinations, and death is its counterpart. Joy is one part of these hallucinations, and misery the other part, and so on.

What have you to do with life or death? These are all creations of the mind. This is called giving up desires of enjoyment either in this life or another.

Then comes controlling the mind, calming it so that it will not break into waves and have all sorts of desires, holding the mind steady, not allowing it to get into waves from external or internal causes, controlling the mind perfectly, just by the power of will. The Jnana-Yogi does not take any one of these physical helps or mental helps: simply philosophic reasoning, knowledge, and his own will, these are the instrumentalities he believes in.

Next comes Titikshâ, forbearance, bearing all miseries without murmuring, without complaining. When an injury comes, do not mind it. If a tiger comes, stand there. Who flies?

There are men who practice Titiksha, and succeed in it. There are men who sleep on the banks of the Ganga in the midsummer sun of India, and in winter float in the waters of the Ganga for a whole day; they do not care. Men sit in the snow of the Himalayas, and do not care to wear any garment. What is heat? What is cold? Let things come and go, what is that to me, I am not the body.

It is hard to believe this in these Western countries, but it is better to know that it is done. Just as your people are brave to jump at the mouth of a cannon, or into the midst of the battlefield, so our people are brave to think and act out their philosophy. They give up their lives for it. "I am Existence-Knowledge-Bliss Absolute; I am He, I am He."

Just as the Western ideal is to keep up luxury in practical life, so ours is to keep up the highest form of spirituality, to demonstrate that religion is riot merely frothy words, but can be carried out, every bit of it, in this life. This is Titiksha, to bear everything, not to complain of anything.

I myself have seen men who say, "I am the soul; what is the universe to me? Neither pleasure nor pain, nor virtue nor vice, nor heat nor cold is anything to me." That is Titiksha; not running after the enjoyments of the body.

What is religion? To pray, "Give me this and that"? Foolish ideas of religion! Those who believe them have no true idea of God and soul. My Master used to say, "The vulture rise higher and higher until he becomes a speck, but his eye is always on the piece of rotten carrion on the earth."

After all, what is the result of your ideas of religion? To cleanse the streets and have more bread and clothes? Who cares for bread and clothes? Millions come and go every minute. Who cares? Why care for the joys and vicissitudes of this little world? Go beyond that if you dare; go beyond law, let the whole universe vanish, and stand alone.

"I am Existence-Absolute, Knowledge-Absolute, Bliss-Absolute; I am He, I am He."

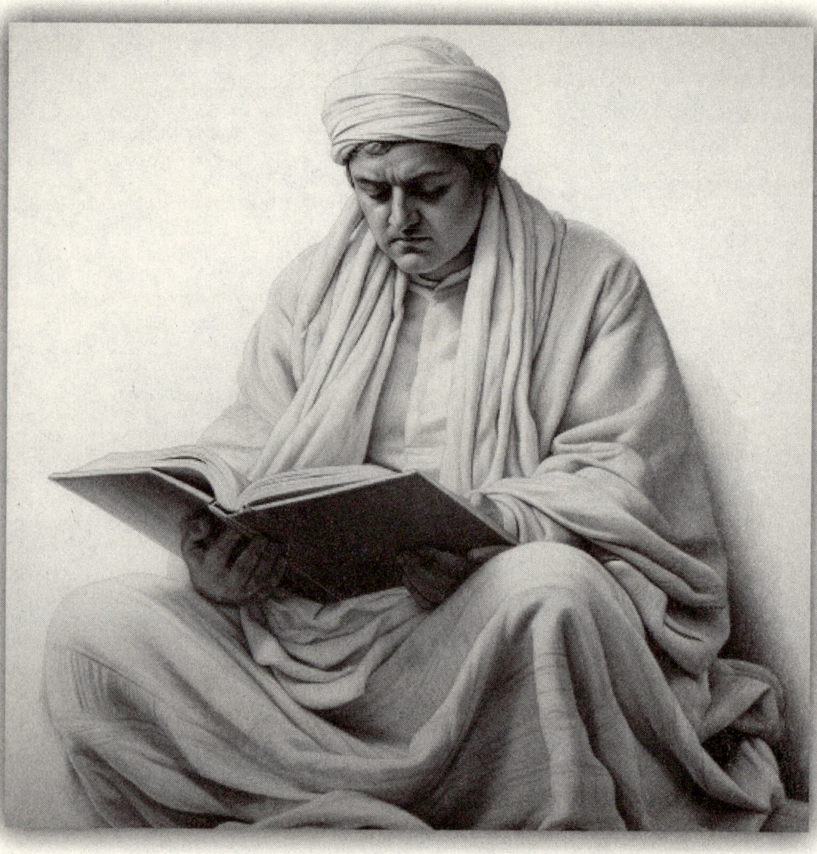

# The Bondage and Freedom Of Atman

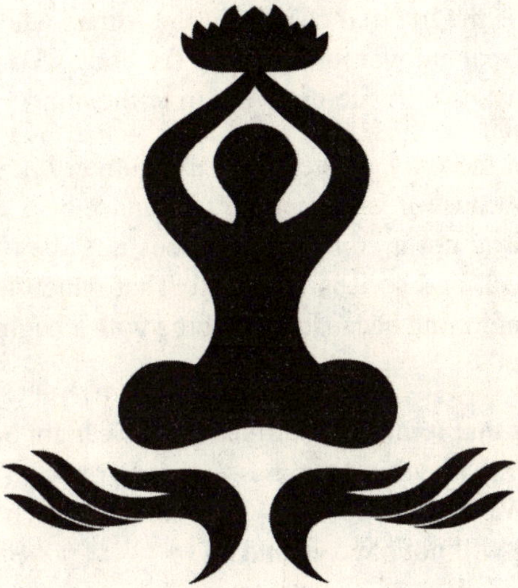

(Delivered in America)

According to the Advaita philosophy, there is only one thing real in the universe, which it calls Brahman; everything else is unreal, manifested and manufactured out of Brahman by the power of Mâyâ. To reach back to that Brahman is our goal. We are, each one of us, that Brahman, that Reality, plus this Maya. If we can get rid of this Maya or ignorance, then we become what we really are.

According to this philosophy, each man consists of three parts — the body, the internal organ or the mind, and behind that, what is called the Âtman, the Self. The body is the external coating and the mind is the internal coating of the Atman who is the real perceiver, the real enjoyer, the being in the body who is working the body by means of the internal organ or the mind.

The Âtman is the only existence in the human body which is immaterial. Because it is immaterial, it cannot be a compound, and because it is not a compound, it does not obey the law of cause and effect, and so it is immortal. That which is immortal can have no beginning because everything with a beginning must have an end.

It also follows that it must be formless; there cannot be any fond without matter. Everything that has form must have a beginning and an end. We have none of us seen a form which had not a beginning and will not have an end.

A form comes out of a combination of force and matter. This chair has a peculiar form, that is to say a certain quantity of matter is acted upon by a certain amount of force and made to assume a particular shape. The shape is the result of a combination of matter and force. The combination cannot be eternal; there must come to every combination a time when it will dissolve.

So all forms have a beginning and an end. We know our body will perish; it had a beginning and it will have an end. But the Self having no form, cannot be bound by the law of beginning and end. It is existing from infinite time; just as time is eternal, so is the Self of man eternal.

Secondly, it must be all-pervading. It is only form that is conditioned and limited by space; that which is formless cannot be confined in space. So, according to Advaita Vedanta, the Self, the Atman, in you, in me, in every one, is omnipresent. You are as much in the sun now as in this earth, as much in England as in America. But the Self acts through the mind and the body, and where they are, its action is visible.

Each work we do, each thought we think, produces an impression, called in Sanskrit Samskâra, upon the mind and the sum total of these impressions becomes the tremendous force which is called "character". The character of a man is what he has created for himself; it is the result of the mental and physical actions that he has done in his life.

The sum total of the Samskaras is the force which gives a man the next direction after death. A man dies; the body falls away and goes back to the elements; but the Samskaras remain, adhering to the mind which, being made of fine material, does not dissolve, because the finer the material, the more persistent it is. But the mind also dissolves in the long run, and that is what we are struggling for.

In this connection, the best illustration that comes to my mind is that of the whirlwind. Different currents of air coming from different directions meet and at the meeting-point become united and go on rotating; as they rotate, they form a body of dust, drawing in bits of paper, straw, etc., at one place, only to drop them and go on to another, and so go on rotating, raising and forming bodies out of the materials which are before them.

Even so the forces, called Prâna in Sanskrit, come together and form the body and the mind out of matter, and move on until the body falls down, when they raise other materials to make another body, and when this falls, another rises, and thus the process goes on. Force cannot travel without matter.

So when the body falls down, the mind-stuff remains, Prana in the form of Samskaras acting on it; and then it goes on to another point, raises up another whirl from fresh materials, and begins another motion. And so it travels from place to place until the force is all spent; and then it falls down, ended.

So when the mind will end, be broken to pieces entirely, without leaving any Samskara, we shall be entirely free, and until that time we are in bondage. Until then the Atman is covered by the whirl of the mind, and imagines it is being taken from place to place.

When the whirl falls down, the Atman finds that It is all-pervading. It can go where It likes, is entirely free, and is able to manufacture any number of minds or bodies It likes; but until then It can go only with the whirl. This freedom is the goal towards which we are all moving.

Suppose there is a ball in this room, and we each have a mallet in our hands and begin to strike the ball, giving it hundreds of blows, driving it from point to point, until at last it flies out of the room. With what force and in what direction will it go out? These will be determined by the forces that have been acting upon it all through the room. All the different blows that have been given will have their effects. Each one of our actions, mental and physical, is such a blow.

The human mind is a ball which is being hit. We are being hit about this room of the world all the time, and our passage out of it is determined by the force of all these blows. In each case, the speed and direction of the ball is determined by the hits it has received; so all our actions in this world will determine our future birth. Our present birth, therefore, is the result of our past.

This is one case: suppose I give you an endless chain, in which there is a black link and a white link alternately, without beginning and without end, and suppose I ask you the nature of the chain. At first you will find a difficulty in determining its nature, the chain being infinite at both ends, but slowly you find out it is a chain. You soon discover that this infinite chain is a repetition of the two links, black and white, and these multiplied infinitely become a whole chain.

If you know the nature of one of these links, you know the nature of the whole chain, because it is a perfect repetition. All our lives, past, present, and future, form, as it were, an infinite chain, without beginning and without end, each link of which is one life, with two ends, birth and death. What we are and do here is being repeated again and again, with but little variation. So if we know these two links, we shall know all the passages we shall have to pass through in this world.

We see, therefore, that our passage into this world has been exactly determined by our previous passages. Similarly we are in this world by our own actions. Just as we go out with the sum total of our present actions upon us, so we see that we come into it with the sum total of our past actions upon us; that which takes us out is the very same thing that brings us in.

What brings us in? Our past deeds. What takes us out? Our own deeds here, and so on and on we go.

Like the caterpillar that takes the thread from its own mouth and builds its cocoon and at last finds itself caught inside the cocoon, we have bound ourselves by our own actions, we have thrown the network of our actions around ourselves. We have set the law of causation in motion, and we find it hard to get ourselves out of it. We have set the wheel in motion, and we are being crushed under it.

So this philosophy teaches us that we are uniformly being bound by our own actions, good or bad.

The Atman never comes nor goes, is never born nor dies. It is nature moving before the Atman, and the reflection of this motion is on the Atman; and the Atman ignorantly thinks it is moving, and not nature. When the Atman thinks that, it is in bondage; but when it comes to find it never moves, that it is omnipresent, then freedom comes.

The Atman in bondage is called Jiva. Thus you see that when it is said that the Atman comes and goes, it is said only for facility of understanding, just as for convenience in studying astronomy you are asked to suppose that the sun moves round the earth, though such is not the case. So the Jiva, the soul, comes to higher or lower states. This is the well-known law of reincarnation; and this law binds all creation.

People in this country think it too horrible that man should come up from an animal. Why? What will be the end of these millions of animals? Are they nothing? If we have a soul, so have they, and if they have none, neither have we. It is absurd to say that man alone has a soul, and the animals none. I have seen men worse than animals.

The human soul has sojourned in lower and higher forms, migrating from one to another, according to the Samskaras or impressions, but it is only in the highest form as man that it attains to freedom. The man form is higher than even the angel form, and of all forms it is the highest; man is the highest being in creation, because he attains to freedom.

All this universe was in Brahman, and it was, as it were, projected out of Him, and has been moving on to go back to the source from which it was projected, like the electricity which comes out of the dynamo, completes the circuit, and returns to it. The same is the case with the soul. Projected from Brahman, it passed through all sorts of vegetable and animal forms, and at last it is in man, and man is the nearest approach to Brahman.

To go back to Brahman from which we have been projected is the great struggle of life. Whether people know it or not does not matter.

In the universe, whatever we see of motion, of struggles in minerals or plants or animals is an effort to come back to the centre and be at rest. There was an equilibrium, and that has been destroyed; and all parts and atoms and molecules are struggling to find their lost equilibrium again.

In this struggle they are combining and re-forming, giving rise to all the wonderful phenomena of nature. All struggles and competitions in animal life, plant life, and everywhere else, all social struggles and wars are but expressions of that eternal struggle to get back to that equilibrium.

The going from birth to death, this travelling, is what is called Samsara in Sanskrit, the round of birth and death literally. All creation, passing through this round, will sooner or later become free.

The question may be raised that if we all shall come to freedom, why should we struggle to attain it? If every one is going to be free, we will sit down and wait. It is true that every being will become free, sooner or later; no one can be lost. Nothing can come to destruction; everything must come up.

If that is so, what is the use of our struggling? In the first place, the struggle is the only means that will bring us to the centre, and in the second place, we do not know why we struggle. We have to.

"Of thousands of men some are awakened to the idea that they will become free." The vast masses of mankind are content with material things, but there are some who awake, and want to get back, who have had enough of this playing, down here. These struggle consciously, while the rest do it unconsciously.

The alpha and omega of Vedanta philosophy is to "give up the world," giving up the unreal and taking the real. Those who are enamoured of the world may ask, "Why should we attempt to get out of it, to go back to the centre? Suppose we have all come from God, but we find this world is pleasurable and nice; then why should we not rather try to get more and more of the world? Why should we try to get out of it?"

They say, look at the wonderful improvements going on in the world every day, how much luxury is being manufactured for it. This is very enjoyable. Why should we go away, and strive for something which is not this?

The answer is that the world is certain to die, to be broken into pieces and that many times we have had the same enjoyments. All the forms which we are seeing now have been manifested again and again, and the world in which we live has been here many times before.

I have been here and talked to you many times before. You will know that it must be so, and the very words that you have been listening to now, you have heard many times before. And many times more it will be the same. Souls were never different, the bodies have been constantly dissolving and recurring.

Secondly, these things periodically occur. Suppose here are three or four dice, and when we throw them, one comes up five, another four, another three, and another two. If you keep on throwing, there must come times when those very same numbers will recur. Go on throwing, and no matter how long may be the interval, those numbers must come again. It cannot be asserted in how many throws they will come again; this is the law of chance.

So with souls and their associations. However distant may be the periods, the same combinations and dissolutions will happen again and again. The same birth, eating and drinking, and then death, come round again and again. Some never find anything higher than the enjoyments of the world, but those who want to soar higher find that these enjoyments are never final, are only by the way.

Every form, let us say, beginning from the little worm and ending in man, is like one of the cars of the Chicago Ferris Wheel which is in motion all the time, but the occupants change. A man goes into a car, moves with the wheel, and comes out. The wheel goes on and on. A soul enters one form, resides in it for a time, then leaves it and goes into another and quits that again for a third. Thus the round goes on till it comes out of the wheel and becomes free.

Astonishing powers of reading the past and the future of a man's life have been known in every country and every age. The explanation is that so long as the Atman is within the realm of causation — though its inherent freedom is not entirely lost and can assert itself, even to the extent of taking the soul out of the causal chain, as it does in the case of men who become free — its actions are greatly influenced by the causal law and thus make it possible for men, possessed with the insight to trace the sequence of effects, to tell the past and the future.

So long as there is desire or want, it is a sure sign that there is imperfection. A perfect, free being cannot have any desire. God cannot want anything. If He desires, He cannot be God. He will be imperfect.

So all the talk about God desiring this and that, and becoming angry and pleased by turns is babies' talk, but means nothing. Therefore it has been taught by all teachers, "Desire nothing, give up all desires and be perfectly satisfied."

A child comes into the world crawling and without teeth, and the old man gets out without teeth and crawling. The extremes are alike, but the one has no experience of the life before him, while the other has gone through it all. When the vibrations of ether are very low, we do not see light, it is darkness; when very high, the result is also darkness. The extremes generally appear to be the same, though one is as distant from the other as the poles.

The wall has no desires, so neither has the perfect man. But the wall is not sentient enough to desire, while for the perfect man there is nothing to desire. There are idiots who have no desires in this world, because their brain is imperfect. At the same time, the highest state is when we have no desires, but the two are opposite poles of the same existence. One is near the animal, and the other near to God.

The mission of the Institute of Thought and Philosophy is to preserve and propagate the teachings of Swami Vivekananda. This great Indian spiritual leader is known for introducing the West to Hinduism. Drawing from his vast literary legacy, we provide valuable insights and practical guidance for modern living.

Have any query or feedback? Please reach out to us at

ITPPress123@gmail.com